THE NEW SCIENCE OF

GRACEFUL AGING

A NEW FRONTIER IN ANTI-AGING THROUGH REGENERATIVE MEDICINE

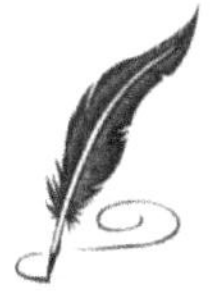

Dr. Farid Rooh, DC, BCIM, CSP

IMPORTANT INFORMATION
FOR THE READER

This information presented in this book has been compiled from my clinical experience and the most up to date research regarding the science of regenerative medicine and overall health and wellness. It is offered as a view of the relationship between regenerative medicine, and health. This book is not intended for, self diagnosis or treatment of disease, nor is it a substitute for the advice and care of a licensed health care provider. Sharing of the information in this book with the attending physician is highly desirable.

This book is intended solely to help you make better judgements concerning your long-term health goals. If you are experiencing health problems or have any specific questions about any medical matter you should consult a qualified physician immediately. If you think you may be suffering from any medical condition you should seek immediate medical attention. You should never delay seeking medical advice, disregard medical advice, or discontinue medical treatment because of information presented in this book

TABLE OF CONTENTS

CHAPTER: 1

WHAT ARE STEM CELLS

What is Stem Cell Therapy?

Stem cells can be defined as undifferentiated cells which have the capacity to proliferate and to differentiate into mature specialized cells (such as brain cells, blood cells, liver cells, etc.). Usage of those stem cells in the field of medicine as a form of therapy is rapidly developing. Many clinical trials and experiments have been done to explore the use of stem/progenitor cells in the treatment of degenerative diseases, different types of cancer and for the repair of damaged or lost tissues. Despite the great promise, there are still many questions regarding the safe application of stem cell therapy (Kehat et al., 2001).

What are the characteristics of Stem Cells?

Since stem cells have the ability to build every tissue in the human body, there is a greater potential therapeutic use for tissue regeneration and repair. To be defined as a "stem cell," a cell must display two essential characteristics. First, it must have the ability of unlimited self-renewal to produce progeny exactly the same as the originating or mother cell. This trait can be seen in cancer cells but those divide in an uncontrolled manner whereas stem cell division is highly regulated(Biehl and Russell, 2009).

Second, under certain physiologic or experimental conditions, it can be induced to become tissue- or organ-specific cells with specialized functions. In some areas of the body, such as the gut or bone marrow, stem cells regularly divide to repair and replace worn out or damaged tissues. In some organs, however, such as the pancreas and the heart, stem cells only divide under special conditions (Ezzone, 2009).

How are Stem Cells formed?

Stem cells are important for living organisms for many reasons. In a 3- to 5-day-old embryo, called a blastocyst, the inner cells give rise to the entire body of the organism, including all of the many specialized cell types and organs such as the heart, skin, or lungs. In some adult tissues, such as bone marrow, muscle, and brain, discrete populations of adult stem cells generate replacements for cells that are lost through normal wear and tear, injury, or disease.

Given their unique regenerative abilities, stem cells offer new potential for treating diseases such as diabetes and heart disease. However, much work needs to be done in laboratory or clinical settings to understand how to use these cells for cell-based therapies to treat disease, an area known as regenerative or reparative medicine.

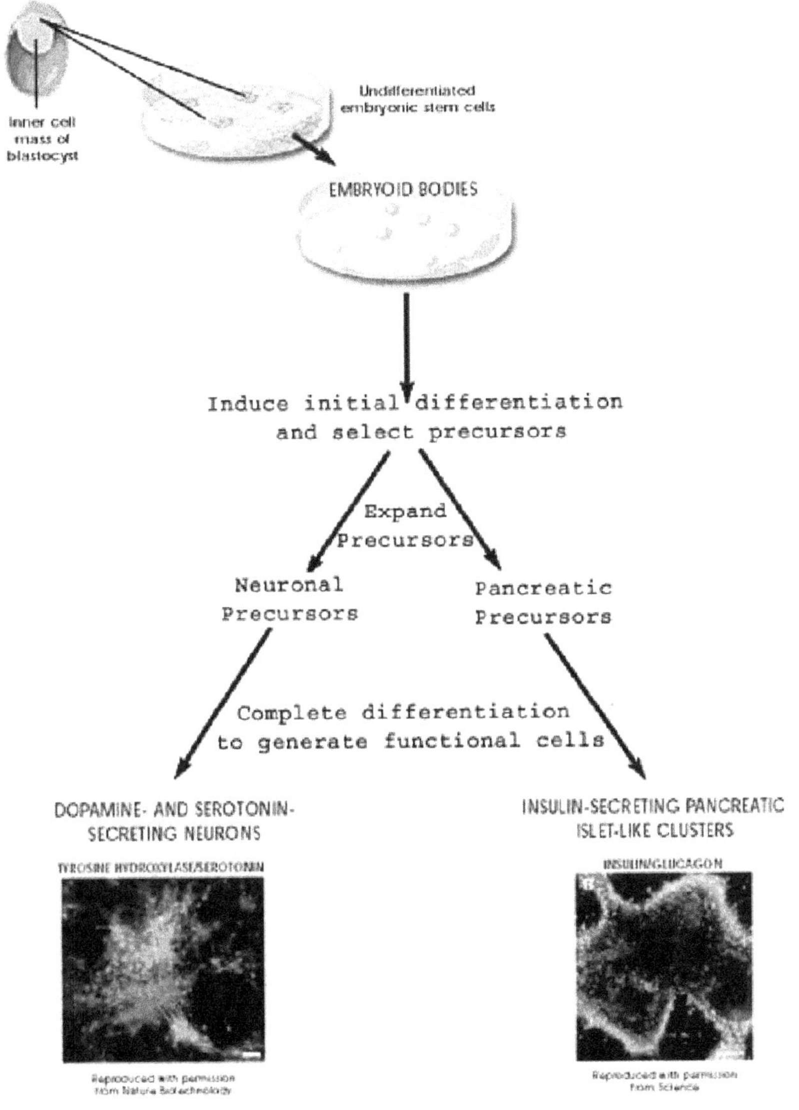

Image 1: Directed differentiation of mouse embryonic stem cells. Image source: Therese Winslow (2008)

Laboratory studies of stem cells enable scientists to figure about the essential properties of cells and what makes them different into other specialized cell types. In fact, many scientists have already been using stem cells in the laboratory to screen new drugs, to develop model systems to study growth and to identify the causes of birth defects (NIH, 2009).

What are Somatic Cells and what types are there?

Until recently, scientists primarily worked with two kinds of stem cells from animals and humans - embryonic stem cells and non-embryonic "adult" or "somatic" stem cells. Scientists identified a number of ways to derive embryonic stem cells from early mouse embryos in 1981. By 1998, the detailed study of the biology of mouse stem cells led to the discovery, of a method to derive stem cells from human embryos and how to grow the cells in the laboratory.

These cells are called human embryonic stem cells. The embryos used in these studies were created for reproductive purposes through *in vitro* fertilization procedures and when they were no longer used for that purpose, they were donated for research with the informed consent of their donor. By 2006, researchers figured out a way to not rely on donated embryos by identifying conditions that would allow some specialized adult cells to be "reprogrammed" genetically to assume a stem cell-like state called induced pluripotent stem cells (IPSCs)(Biehl and Russell, 2009).

Stem cells are important for living organisms for many reasons. In the blastocyst, the inner cells give rise to the entire body of the organism. In older tissues, adult stem cells generate replacements for cells that are lost through normal wear and tear, injury, or disease (Biehl and Russell, 2009).

Apart from humans and animals, plant stem cells have also been discovered. Plant stem cells are innately undifferentiated cells located in the meristems of plant which are capable of giving rise to a steady supply of precursor cells to form differentiated tissues and organs in the plant (Shen et al., 2013).

Just as there are many different types of specialized or differentiated cells in the body, there are many different types of stem cells in the body. Hierarchically, stem cells are classified as totipotent, pluripotent, multipotent, and unipotent.

Pluripotent stem cells are so named because they have the ability to differentiate into all cell types in the body. In natural development, pluripotent stem cells are only present for a very short period of time in the embryo before differentiating into the more specialized multipotent stem cells that eventually give rise to the specialized tissues of the body. These more limited multipotent stem cells come in several subtypes: some can become only cells of a particular germ line (endoderm, mesoderm, ectoderm) and others, only cells of a particular tissue. In other words, pluripotent cells can eventually become any cell of the body by differentiating into multipotent stem cells that go through a series of divisions into even more restricted specialized cells.

The most plastic type of stem cells which have the capability to theoretically give rise to any possible cell type including the entire organism are called totipotent. Two examples are the zygote and oocyte.

In the end, where the plasticity of stem cells end, the non-plastic version of cells known as unipotent cell types begin .Such cells are not stem cells, but are rather somatic cells and these are the majority of cell types in the human body. These cells are capable of dividing and giving rise to only their own cell type. A typical example are the glial cells found within the nervous system which can give rise to only other glial cells. So, broadly speaking the basic types of stem cells can be divided as embryonic and adult/ somatic stem cells. Also, their sources are so called from embryonic origin (mostly totipotent and pluripotent stem cells) and somatic tissue (adult stem cells like-hematopoietic stemcells, muscle stem cells, liver stem cells etc.) respectively.

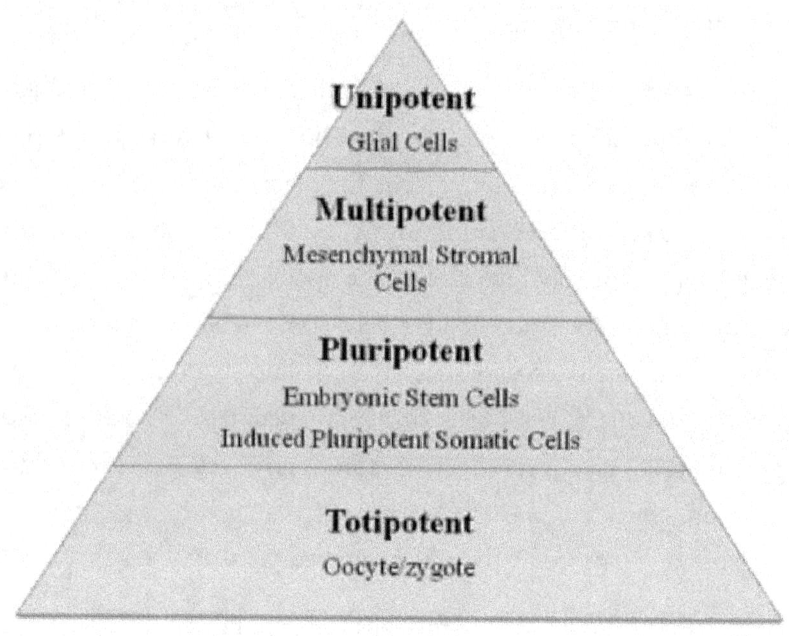

Image source: (Ezzone, 2009)

SOURCES OF STEM CELLS

Embryonic Stem Cells (ES)

Embryonic stem cells are derived from the embryo. They are derived 7-10 days after fertilization from the pre-implantation blastocyst and as mentioned above, ES cells are Pluripotent. Ethical considerations have prompted into other stem cell research sources because deriving ES cells disrupts the Blastocyst. (NIH, 2015)

How Embroyonic stem cells are grown?

Human embryonic stem cells (hESCs) are generated by transferring cells from a pre-implantation stage embryo into a plastic laboratory culture dish that contains a nutrient broth known as culture medium where the cells divide and spread over the surface of the dish. In the original protocol, the inner surface of the culture dish was coated with mouse embryonic skin cells specially treated so they will not divide. This coating layer of cells is called a feeder layer. The mouse cells in the bottom of the culture dish provide the cells a sticky surface to which they can attach. Also, the feeder cells release nutrients into the culture medium. Researchers have now devised ways to grow embryonic stem cells without mouse feeder cells. This is a significant scientific advance because of the risk that viruses or other macromolecules in the mouse cells may be transmitted to the human cells.(NIH, 2015)

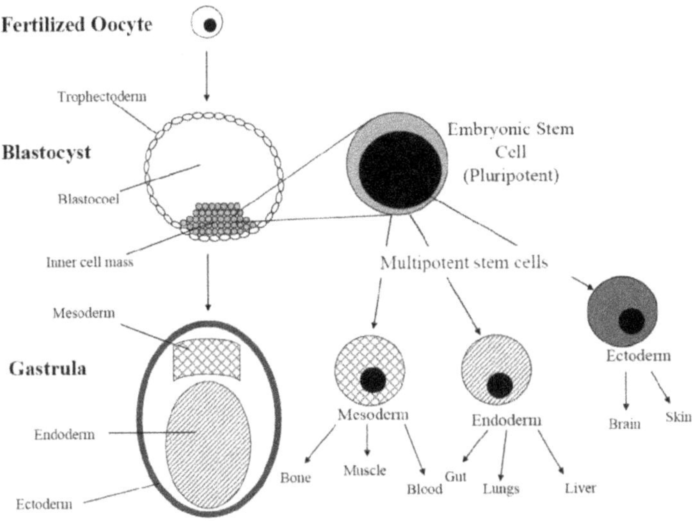

Derivation of Stem cells (Biehl and Russell, 2009).

The process of generating an embryonic stem cell line is somewhat inefficient, so lines that are not producing each time cells from the pre-implantation stage embryo are placed into a culture dish. However, if the plated cells survive, divide and multiply enough to crowd the dish, they are removed gently and plated into several fresh culture dishes. The process of re-plating or sub culturing the cells is repeated many times and for many months.

Each cycle of sub culturing the cells is referred to as a passage; Once the cell line is established, the original cells yield millions of embryonic stem cells. Embryonic stem cells that have proliferated in cell culture for six or more months without differentiating, are pluripotent, and appear genetically normal are referred to as an embryonic stem cell line; At any stage in the process, batches of cells can be frozen and shipped to other laboratories for further culture and experimentation.(NIH, 2015)

Adult Stem Cells

Adult stem cells, also known as somatic stem cells, are present in most, but not all tissues. They are mostly multipotent, however pluripotent adult stem cells exist in small number. They persist throughout life and possess the role of maintaining and repairing tissue, in which they are found, in response to injury. They have been identified in many tissues including brain, bone marrow, blood vessels, heart, liver, and others. They reside in a specific area of each tissue called a stem cell niche(NIH, 2015).

Induced Pluripotent Stem Cells (IPS)

An experiment was done in 2006 to figure out which genes that were usually expressed in embryonic stem cells were introduced into mature somatic cells. This process, called reprogramming, lead a small number of mature cells to revert back to a highly immature cell state that resembled an embryonic stem cell. It induced a pluripotent state in a previously differentiated cell, hence the name (NIH, 2015).

History of Stem Cell Usage:

The early 1900's European researchers realized that the various type of blood cells - white blood cells, red blood cells and platelets - all came from a particular 'stem cell'. However, it was only in 1963 that the first quantitative descriptions of the self-renewing activities of transplanted mouse bone marrow stem cells were documented by Canadian researchers,

Ernest A McCulloch and James E Til (Mcculloch, Till and Becker, 1963).

Then, in 1998, James Thomson, a scientist at the University of Wisconsin in Madison, successfully removed cells from spare embryos at fertility clinics and grew them in the laboratory. This launched stem cell research into the limelight, establishing the world's first human embryonic stem cell line which still exists today (Thomson, 1998).

Early studies of mouse embryos in 1981 by two researchers at Cambridge University, M. J. Evans and M. H. Kaufman, established a platform for pluripotent stem cells (Evans and Kaufman, 1981). The breakthrough discovery came when artificial counterparts of natural pluripotent stem cells were generated in a dish by Shinya Yamanaka and his group from Japan in 2007. Yamanaka's group demonstrated for the first time that by introducing four pluripotency genes named Oct4, Sox2, Klf4 and c-Myc, somatic cells can be made to behave like pluripotent stem cells. The stem cells generated by this method were termed as Induced Pluripotent stem cells (iPSC)(Yamanaka, 2007).

Then onwards, the standard technology for generating iPSCs have been used globally to generate pluripotent stem cells from various cell types and used in basic science research as well as the applied aspect of stem cell biology.

This timeline takes you through the history of the stem cell therapy:

1981, Mouse beginnings

Embryonic stem cells – in mice by Martin Evans of Cardiff University, UK, at the University of Cambridge, is first to identify (UNMC, 2018).

1997, Dolly the sheep

Ian Wilmut and his colleagues at the Roslin Institute, Edinburgh unveiled Dolly the sheep, the first artificial animal clone. The process involves fusing a sheep egg with an udder cell and implanting the resulting hybrids into a surrogate mother sheep. Researchers speculate that similar hybrids made by fusing human embryonic stem cells with adult cells from a particular person could be used to create genetically matched tissue and organs which made a huge controversy(UNMC, 2018).

1998, Stem cells go human

James Thomson of the University of Wisconsin in Madison and John Gearhart of Johns Hopkins University in Baltimore, respectively, isolate human embryonic stem cells and grow them in the lab(UNMC, 2018).

2001, Bush controversy

U.S. President George W. Bush limits federal funding of research on human embryonic stem cells because a human embryo is destroyed in the process. But President Bush does allow continued research on human embryonic stem cells lines that were created before the restrictions were announced(UNMC, 2018).

2005, Fraudulent clones

Woo Suk Hwang of Seoul National University in South Korea reports that his team has used therapeutic cloning – a technique inspired by the one used to create Dolly – to create human embryonic stem cells genetically matched to specific people. Later that year, his claims turn out to be false(UNMC, 2018).

2006, Cells reprogrammed

Shinya Yamanaka of Kyoto University in Japan reveals a way of making embryonic-like cells from adult cells – avoiding the need to destroy an embryo. His team reprograms ordinary adult cells by inserting four key genes – forming "induced pluripotent stem cells".

2007, Nobel prize

Evans shares the Nobel prize for medicine with Mario Capecchi and Oliver Smithies for work on genetics and embryonic stem cells.

2009, Obama changes

President Barack Obama lifts 2001 restrictions on federal funding for human embryonic stem cell research.

2010, Spinal injury

A person with spinal injury becomes the first to receive a medical treatment derived from human embryonic stem cells as part of a trial by Geron of Menlo Park, California, a pioneering company for human embryonic stem cell therapies(UNMC, 2018).

2012, Blindness treated

Human embryonic stem cells show medical promise in a treatment that eases blindness(UNMC, 2018).

2012, Another Nobel

Yamanaka wins a Nobel prize for creating induced pluripotent stem cells, which he shares with John Gurdon of the University of Cambridge.

2013, Therapeutic cloning

Shoukhrat Mitalipov at the Oregon National Primate Research Center in Beaverton and his colleagues produce human embryonic stem cells from fetal cells using therapeutic cloning – the breakthrough falsely claimed in 2005(UNMC, 2018).

2014, Pre-embryonic state

Charles Vacanti of Harvard Medical School together with Haruko Obokata at the Riken Center for Developmental Biology in Kobe, Japan, and colleagues announced a revolutionary discovery that any cell can potentially be rewound to a pre-embryonic state – using a simple, 30-

minute technique(UNMC, 2018).

2014, Therapeutic cloning – with adult cells

Teams led by Dieter Egli of the New York Stem Cell Foundation and Young Gie Chung from CHA University in Seoul, South Korea, independently produce human embryonic stem cells from adult cells, using therapeutic cloning. Egli's team use skin cells from a woman with diabetes and demonstrate that the resulting stem cells can be turned into insulin-producing beta cells. In theory, the cells could be used to replace those lost to the disease(UNMC, 2018).

2014, Human trials

Masayo Takahashi at the same Riken centre is due to select patients for what promises to be the world's first trial of a therapy based on induced pluripotent stem cells, to treat a form of age-related blindness (UNMC, 2018).

Usage of Stem Cell Therapy/ Advantages

There are many ways in which human stem cells can be used in research and the clinic. These research studies will yield information about the complex events that occur during human development. One of the main goals of this work is to identify the mechanism of undifferentiated stem cells becoming the differentiated cells that form the tissues and organs all over the body.

So far scientists have figured out that alteration or basically the mutations of genes is central to this process where medical conditions, such as cancer and birth defects have been identified are due to abnormal cell division and differentiation. A more complete understanding of the genetic and molecular mechanisms such as cell death pathways and related enzymes etc may yield information about how such diseases arise and suggest new strategies for therapy. The recent developments with iPS cells suggest some of the specific factors that may be involved, techniques must be devised to introduce these factors safely into the cells and control the processes that are induced by these factors(Ezzone, 2009).

Human stem cells are currently being used to test new drugs. Newly invented medications are tested for safety on differentiated cells generated from human pluripotent cell lines before introducing it as a proper drug to the Market. Other kinds of cell lines have a long history of being used in this way. Cancer cell lines, for example, are used to screen potential anti-tumor drugs. The availability of pluripotent stem cells would allow drug testing in a wider range of cell types(NIH, 2009).

However, to screen drugs effectively and more accurately the conditions especially the stem cell differentiation must be identical when comparing different drugs. Therefore, scientists are currently looking on to precisely controlling the differentiation of stem cells into the specific cell type on which drugs will be tested. Current knowledge of the signals controlling cell differentiation lags behind which need to figure out cells being able to mimic these conditions precisely to generate pure populations of differentiated cells for each drug being tested(NIH, 2009).

Cell-based therapies perhaps the most important potential application of human stem cells is the generation of cells and tissues that could be used. Today, donated organs and tissues are often used to replace ailing or destroyed tissue, but the need for transplantable tissues and organs far outweighs the available supply. Stem cells, directed to differentiate into specific cell types, offer the possibility of a renewable source of replacement cells and tissues to treat diseases including Alzheimer's disease, spinal cord injury, stroke, burns, heart disease, diabetes, osteoarthritis, and rheumatoid arthritis(NIH, 2009).

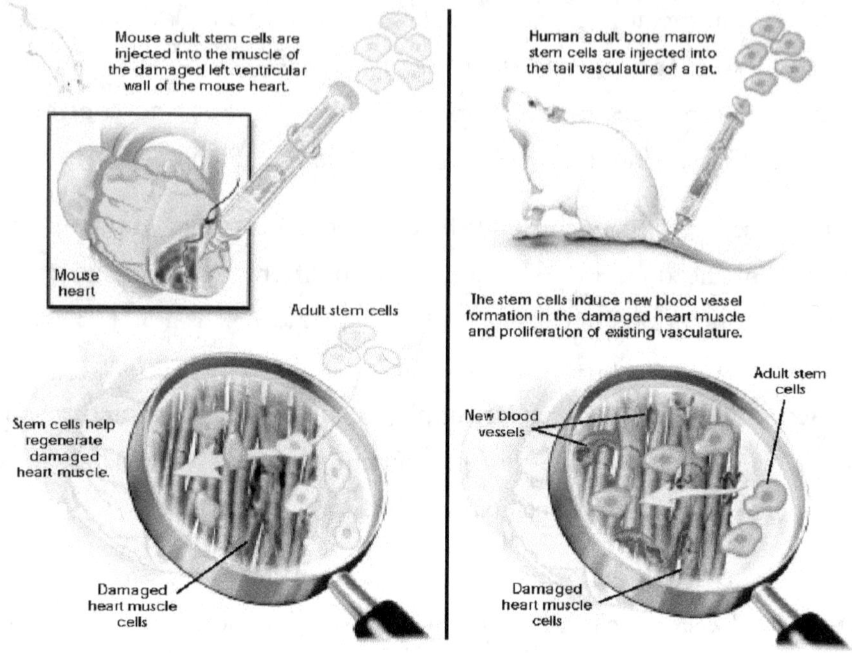

Image Source: (NIH, 2009) Image source: Therese Winslow (2008)

It has figured out that there is a possibility to generate healthy heart muscle cells in the laboratory and then transplant those cells into patients with chronic heart disease. Preliminary research in mice and other animals indicates that bone marrow stromal cells, transplanted into a damaged heart, can have beneficial effects. Whether these cells can generate heart muscle cells or stimulate the growth of new blood vessels that repopulate the heart tissue, or help via some other mechanism is actively under investigation.

For example, rather than actually incorporating into the heart, injected cells may repair by secreting growth factors. Promising results from cell culture systems indicate that it may be possible to direct the differentiation of embryonic stem cells or adult bone marrow cells into heart muscle cells(NIH, 2009).

Risk Factors Associated in STM.

Risks associated with stem cell therapy depend on many risk factors. A risk is defined as a combination of the probability of occurrence of harm and the severity of that harm(Perin, Geng and Willerson, 2003).

Examples of risk factors are the type of stem cells used, their procurement and culturing history, the level of manipulation and site of injection. Because of the variety of risk factors, the risks associated with different stem cell based medicinal products may differ widely as well. For an adequate benefit/risk assessment of a stem cell based medicinal product, all important identified risks (i.e. risks or adverse events identified in clinical experience) as well as potential/theoretical risks (e.g. non-clinical safety concerns) that have not been observed in clinical experience should be thoroughly evaluated (Herberts, Kwa and Hermsen, 2011).

Such an evaluation at the start and during the development of a stem cell based therapy may help to determine the extent and focus of the product development and safety evaluation plans. Overview of the risk factors are shown in the table below.

Factors	Risk factors or Hazard	Identified Risk
Intrinsic factors Cell Characteristics:	Origin of cells (e.g. autologous vs. allogenic, diseased vs. healthy donor/tissue) Differentiation status - - Tumourigenic potential - Proliferation capacity - Life span - Long term viability - Excretion patterns (e.g. growth factors, cytokines, chemokines)	Disease susceptibility- Unwanted biological effect (e.g. in vivo differentiation in unwanted cell type) Toxicity- Neoplasm formation (benign or malignant)
Extrinsic factors Manufacturing and handling	Lack of donor history - - Starting and raw materials - - Plasma derived materials - Mix-up of autologous patient material	Disease transmission Reactivation of latent viruses

	Cell handling procedures (e.g. procurement) - - Culture duration - Tumourigenic potential (e.g. culture induced transformation, incomplete removal of undifferentiated cells) - Non cellular components - Pooling of allogenic cell populations - Conservation (e.g. cryopreservatives) - Storage conditions (e.g. failure of traceability, human material labelling) - Transport conditions	Cell line contamination (e.g. with unwanted cells, growth media components, chemicals) Contamination by adventitious agents (viral/bacterial/ mycoplasma/fungi, prions, parasites) Neoplasm formation (benign or malignant)

Clinical characteristics	Therapeutic use (i.e. homologous or non-homologous) - - Indication - - Administration route - - Initiation of immune responses - Use of immune supressives - Exposure duration - Underlying disease - Irreversibility of the treatment	Undesired immune response (e.g. GVHD) Unintended physiological and anatomical consequences (e.g. arrhythmia) Engraftment at unwanted location Toxicity Lack of efficacy neoplasm formation (benign or malignant)

Source: (Herberts, Kwa and Hermsen, 2011)

CHAPTER: 2

THE HISTORY OF

REGENERATIVE MEDICINE.

When were stem cells discovered?

Stem cells were first discovered by Canadian scientists James Till and Earnest McCulloch, in 1963. The two were experimenting with a bone marrow transplant in irradiated mice when they made the discovery.

Who was involved in the beginning?

Till and McCulloch noticed the changes in the mice spleens. Little lumps were forming on them. They found it interesting that the number of lumps correlated with the number of transplanted bone marrow cells (1 lump for every 10.000 cells). Till and McCulloch correctly recognized these were cell colonies. They were helped in their research by Dr. Lou Siminovitch and a graduate student Andy Becker. These two concluded, after studying the colonies, that they were formed by clone cells who could self-renew. What they discovered were blood-forming stem cells.

What is a stem cell?

A stem cell is a type of cell that can change into another type of cell through a process called cellular differentiation. This means that a stem cell can become a muscle cell, bone cell, immune cell, blood cell, nervous cell, fat cell, etc. When stem cells differentiate and become adult cells of another type, they can divide and create more cells of the same type. Humans and all mammals have two basic types of stem cells. These are embryonic stem cells and adult, or somatic, stem cells.

What is a Mesenchymal Stem Cell (MSC)?

Mesenchymal stem cells (MSC) are multipotent connective tissue cells. MSC can differentiate into several cell types, such as bone cells, muscle cells, fat cells, etc. The name, mesenchymal stem cell, is derived from mesenchyme, a type of embryonic connective tissue. MSC's are found in the bone marrow, umbilical cord, body fat (adipose tissue), and amniotic fluid. These cells are a subject of many studies because of their accessibility and potential therapeutic properties. Scientists believe that MSC's could be used in the treatment of orthopedic injuries, autoimmune diseases, cardiovascular diseases, liver diseases, and graft versus host disease (N. Kim, S. Cho, 2013).

What are induced pluripotent stem cells (iPS)?

Pluripotent stem cells are stem cells that can differentiate (change) into any of the three primary cell layers, the so-called germ layers (endoderm, mesoderm, and ectoderm). Therefore, pluripotent stem cells have the potential to differentiate into many other cell types. However, only embryonic stem cells are pluripotent while adult stem cells are not. This was a big ethical problem for researchers because the generation of these cells requires manipulation, and often destruction, of the human embryo. In 2006, Japanese scientist Shinya Yamanaka found a way to convert adult cells into pluripotent stem cells. These were named induced pluripotent stem cells (iPS). Mr. Yamanaka received a Nobel Prize in 2012 for his breakthrough discovery. Induced pluripotent stem cells have great therapeutic potential. They can be derived directly from the patient's tissue, personalizing each treatment. Induced pluripotent stem cells are grown in the laboratory using human donor cells induced with four stem cell-associated genes. As a result, some of the donor cells become iPS cells and can be harvested and cultivated for further use (S. Yamanaka, 2012).

What is cell potency?

According to their ability to change into other cell types, cells can be totipotent, pluripotent, multipotent, oligopotent, and unipotent. Cells with greater potency can differentiate into more cell types. Totipotent cells, such as spores and zygotes, can differentiate into all cell types found in a certain organism. Pluripotent cells, like embryonic stem cells in humans, can differentiate in many other cell types. Multipotent cells can differentiate into related cell types. For example, connective tissue stem cells can differentiate into other connective tissue cell types. Oligopotent cells can differentiate into a few closely related cell types while unipotent cells can differentiate into only one cell type. The existence of true unipotent cells is still a matter of scientific debate (T.S. Macfarlane et al. 2012).

Autologous harvesting and its origins?

Autologous harvest of stem cells is the process of collecting blood-forming stem cells from the patients' bloodstream. The cells harvested in this way are referred to as peripheral blood stem cells (PBSC's). These cells are used in cancer treatment to replace the blood-forming cells killed by chemotherapy, along with cancer cells. Autologous stem cell harvesting was developed to enable stem cell transplants for people who had no matching donors. American scientist E. Donnell Thomas pioneered stem cell transplantation in the 1950s, eventually winning a Nobel Prize in Physiology and Medicine (I. Henig, T. Zuckerman, 2014).

Why do organ transplants have immune rejection?

The main function of the immune system is to protect from harmful "foreign bodies" such as bacteria, viruses, cancer cells, etc. The immune system recognizes those foreign bodies by special proteins called antigens located on their surface. All people have different antigens so all transplanted tissues are recognized as foreign bodies by the immune system and rejected to a certain level. However, the donor's and the recipient's tissues can be closely matched. In such cases, transplantation can be successful. When they are not well-matched, acute or chronic rejection of the transplanted tissue occurs (A. Moreau, et al. 2013).

How do organ transplants relate to regenerative medicine?

Organ transplants and regenerative medicine have a lot in common. These two disciplines complement each other. Right now, organ transplants are still the best and often the only option for people in need of organ replacement. The ultimate goal of regenerative medicine, in the future, is to offer to the patients' new organs and tissues made from their cells. At this moment, organ transplants are still risky procedures. Rejection of transplanted tissue remains a big issue. Regenerative medicine has the potential to offer repairs of damaged organs, to restore their function and avoid the need for transplantation (G. Orlando, et al. 2013).

What are the embryonic stem cells and umbilical stem

cells? What are the differences between them?

Embryonic stem cells and umbilical stem cells differ significantly. The first major difference is in their potency. Embryonic stem cells are pluripotent, which means that they can differentiate into most other cell types. This gives embryotic cells a potentially much wider field of application. Umbilical stem cells are multipotent. They are blood stem cells that can differentiate into other types of blood cells, including immune cells. Another important difference is their availability. Embryonic stem cells are harvested only from the human embryo, before its implantation. This method raises many ethical questions and restrains scientific research about embryonic stem cells and their use. Umbilical stem cells are much more available because they are harvested from the blood located in the umbilical cord, a resource previously discarded as medical waste (M. Weiss, D. Troyer, 2006).

What makes stem cells different from other cells?

All stem cells have three major characteristics that make them different from other cells. Firstly, stem cells can divide and renew themselves for a long time. This process is often referred to as cell proliferation. Secondly, unlike other cells, stem cells are not specialized. Thirdly, stem cells are very potent. They can change (differentiate) into almost all specialized cell types (NIH, 2019).

What are the controversies, ethical and moral issues regarding the use of embryonic tissue for research?

Stem cells are often a subject of controversy, mainly because of some ethical concerns about embryonic stem cell research. The common misconceptions that cause these controversies are the alleged use of aborted fetuses for stem cell research and the manipulation with the human embryo. The first claim is completely false. Embryonic stem cell do not and cannot come from aborted fetuses. They can only be harvested from a 4 to 5 days old non-implanted human embryo. This leads us to the second controversy which requires an answer to the following question. Are human embryos destroyed during the process? The answer is yes. However, these are non-implanted human embryos. They are donated by In Vitro Fertilization clinics because they are already destined for destruction for various reasons.

Why has it taken the USA so long to catch up to the other countries?

The main reason for the USA falling behind in stem cell research is the government-imposed restriction on federal funding. In 1996 the Dickey-Wicker amendment was passed in Congress banning federal funding of any research activity that can cause harm to human embryos. The biggest drawback, however, happened in 2001 when President George W. Bush banned federal funding of any newly created embryonic stem cell lines. Since then the legislation was loosened up a bit, especially under the Obama presidency.

What does the USA medical community think about it?

A prevailing opinion in the medical community is that the United States has to do more if they want to remain competitive in the field of stem cell research. Coordinated actions of universities, legislators, private entities, etc. are thought to be necessary. Scientists recognize the potential and hope that stem cell research brings for the treatment of a great number of diseases.

Could this be the future answer to organ transplants and donations?

Stem cells are a very promising future solution for organ and tissue repair. Theoretically, it could even become possible to create brand new organs using stem cells. More research is necessary but regenerative medicine has plenty of potentials to completely replace organ transplants in the future.

How can IVF assist in harvesting stem cells?

In Vitro Fertility clinics store non-implanted human embryos. In certain cases, these embryos are deemed unfit for implantation and have to be discarded. In such cases, IVF clinics can decide to donate these embryos for embryonic stem cell research with the informed consent of the donor. Also, couples or individuals who decide that they do not want to store their embryos in IVF clinics anymore can choose to donate them for scientific research. Therefore, IVF clinics can be a very valuable source of research material.

Are embryonic stem cells used clinically to treat disease?

Despite their promising potential, embryonic stem cells found only a limited and largely experimental clinical application. Scientists are aware that stem cell use in medical treatment could potentially result in the development of an effective treatment for various diseases, including Parkinson's disease and cancer. Stem cells also have the potential to revolutionize organ replacement and tissue repair. However, except for the hematopoietic stem cell transplantation (bone marrow transplantation), stem cell therapy has not had much clinical success yet (J. Poulos, 2018).

How has Dolly, the famous sheep cloning from a stem cell line, helped the advance of regenerative medicine since 1996?

Cloning of Dolly the sheep was a breakthrough in genetic engineering and an important point in stem cell research. Scientists who took part in this project proved that it is possible to reprogram a fully developed adult cell and turn it into a newly-fertilized embryo. This encouraged other researchers to look for ways to reprogram adult cells and eventually led to the creation of the induced pluripotent stem cells (I. Wilmut, et al. 2009).

Can regenerative medicine offer a way to cure disease and not merely treat the symptoms and revolutionize modern medicine?

To treat the disease rather than just symptoms is the promise on which regenerative medicine is yet to deliver. Regenerative medicine has the potential to revolutionize disease treatment. By being able to replace the damaged cells and tissues regenerative medicine could, for example, repair the brain of patients with Parkinson's instead of only trying to control the tremors and other symptoms. The same goes for almost all other diseases such as diabetes, cardiovascular diseases, cancer, etc. Regenerative medicine will make it possible to use the healing powers of our bodies to completely cure these diseases, in the future.

Can embryonic stem cell transplants cause tumors?

There are two different cancer risks related to stem cell transplants. The first one is the possibility of cancer relapse. When the cancer returns after the stem cell transplant treatment, new stem cell transplant is rarely possible. The development of new cancer after stem cell transplant procedure is also possible but rare. However, scientists believe that the risk is associated with the type of transplant and the type of stem cells used. According to this, higher risk of cancer development is associated with allogeneic transplants (donor stem cells) and with embryonic stem cells because of their high proliferation rate (C.A. Herberts, et al. 2011).

Where are stem cells found in the body and the different types found in each area?

Embryonic stem cells are found only in 3 to 5 days old blastocysts. A blastocyst resembles a small ball of cells. It is a young human embryo. Adult stem cells can be found in different tissues throughout the body. These are multipotent tissue-specific cells. Scientists have found them in the bone marrow, blood, blood vessels, liver, skin, skeletal muscles, brain, and heart. Normally, adult stem cells located in a certain type of tissue can differentiate into many similar cell types. Mesenchymal cells, for example, are connective tissue cells that can differentiate into bone, cartilage, and fat cells among others (NIH, 2019).

Can the transplants of stem cells get immune rejected?

Recipients' immune system can sometimes reject donors' stem cells after transplant. This is a rare complication and it can usually be treated with a new transplant. Another stem cell transplant-related complication, opposite of rejection, can be much more serious. It is called the graft versus host disease (GvHD). This is a condition in which the newly formed blood cells, created by the donors' stem cells, recognize the host's cells as foreign bodies and attack them. (R. Zeiser, B. Blazar, 2017).

In 1968 the first bone marrow transplant occurred, 1981 the first stem cell in vitro cell line was developed, stem cells in the placenta were discovered in 2007, in 2016 we are using stem cells clinically to treat degenerative diseases. What will be next?

Medical and scientific communities, as well as the greater public, have great hopes and expectation of stem cell research in the future. Many experts believe that stem cells are the future of medicine. The ongoing research will provide even more knowledge. The applications of stem cells in medicine will be numerous in the future. Stem cells will make it possible to slow down the aging process and reduce its effects. We will be able to regenerate all tissues and cure diseases such as Parkinson's and diabetes. It might even become possible to produce new organs and tissues from patients' cells and replace the malfunctioning ones (UK Academy of Sciences, 2018).

Why do we heal slower when we are older?

Wounds heal slower in older individuals because the coordinated effort of various cells required for healing slows down. The level of communication between these cells also becomes lower. For example, human skin needs skin cells (keratinocytes) and immune cells to work together during healing. Keratinocytes communicate with the immune cells throughout the process, signaling to them to help. In younger people, this process is smooth and takes less time. Keratinocytes of older people do not migrate fast enough to the area of the wound and do not produce enough signals to communicate with immune cells successfully (Rockefeller University, 2016).

How do we rejuvenate "old" tissue?

In theory, tissue repair and rejuvenation can best be achieved with the use of some kind of stem cell therapy. Pluripotent stem cells have the potential to replace almost all types of aging cells. With their proliferation ability, repair of "old" tissue should be simple. In reality, things are far more complicated. There are many factors, such as lifestyle, environment, chronic, and degenerative diseases, that influence the process of aging. Even the properties of stem cells are affected by aging. Scientists are aware that it will take more time and research to understand and overcome all the obstacles in this process (J. Neves, et al. 2017).

How does a stem cell age and what does it do while it ages?

Stem cells can age too. The aging process affects all of stem cells' characteristics. Their ability to differentiate into other cell types is changed gradually over time. Stem cells also lose their renewal ability with age. Scientists are still researching how the aging of the stem cells affects the aging process in general (A.S. Ahmed, et al. 2017).

What is an adult stem cell (ASC) and where are they found?

Most cells that form tissue or an organ are specialized cells (e.g. muscle cells in muscles, blood cells in the blood, etc.). However, some cells have not yet developed (differentiated) into a specialized cell type. We refer to them as undifferentiated cells or adult stem cells. The main role of these cells is to repair the tissue in which they are found. They do this by changing into other cell types and creating new cells of the same specialized type. Adult stem cells can be found in many tissues and organs, including bone marrow, umbilical cord blood, heart, brain, intestines, testicles, mammary glands, etc. Adult stem cells from bone marrow have been used in clinical treatment for more than 40 years (NIH, 2019).

What is an amniotic fluid-derived stem cell (AFSC)? When did this discovery occur?

Amniotic fluid stem cells (AFSC) are several types of multipotent cells derived from amniotic fluid. The two most important stem cell types found in the amniotic fluid are mesenchymal stem cells and embryonic-like stem cells. These cells can differentiate into several specialized tissue cells, such as bone, cartilage, muscle, nerves, skin, and cardiac tissue. Because of this AFSC's could potentially be used for organ regeneration. AFSC's were discovered in 2007 by the research team of Dr. Anthony Atala at the Institute for Regenerative Medicine at Wake Forest University in Winston-Salem, N.C. (A. Atala, et al. 2009).

What is an extracellular matrix? How is it used in regenerative medicine?

In science, the term extracellular refers to the molecules located outside of the cell. These are commonly molecules of collagen, elastin, other proteins, and enzymes. The extracellular matrix is a network of such molecules, a three-dimensional one. Many cells bind to the extracellular matrix. This promotes healing of tissue. That is why the extracellular matrix is used in regenerative medicine, especially in tissue engineering. Here, the extracellular matrix is used as a kind of scaffolding on which the cells are cultivated to enable functional reconstruction of various tissue types (S. Yi, et al. 2017).

How can lifestyle factors affect stem cells?

Different lifestyle factors can affect stem cells. One study shows that type 2 diabetes can change the regenerative potential of mesenchymal stem cells. Researchers from MIT have discovered a connection between gut health and stem cell properties. They've concluded that fasting can improve the ability of stem cells to regenerate. Long-term exposure to inflammation can seriously compromise bone marrow transplants (hematopoietic stem cells), by exhausting the stem cells and slowing their proliferation. (C. Kizil, et al. 2015).

What gets in the way of healing?

Chronic diseases such as diabetes, bad blood circulation, weak immune system, unhealthy diet, infections, smoking, chemotherapy, radiation, and other factors can negatively affect the healing process.

What assists healing?

Healing is a natural process that involves tissue repair and happens on a cellular level. That is why stem cells have a very positive effect on healing. Other factors can help the process of healing, such as lifestyle and environmental factors. A healthy diet, physical activity, and non-smoking are just some of the examples.

CHAPTER: 3

THE CURRENT STATE OF PAIN AND ITS GRIP ON AMERICA

Chronic diseases are the number one money maker for the medical industry. Treating patients with heart disease, cancer, diabetes and musculoskeletal pain is what the medical industry does. It's where medicine makes its money. We are constantly looking through research for ways to mess with the genome to "fix" our broken genetics. By altering and treating these screwed up blueprints (our genes) of life we could fix chronic disease. However, after trillions of dollars and decades of research we consistently show that lifestyle is more important than the genes within us. Interfering with the genome will find ways to potentially treat something but a real cure eludes us. We are not addressing true healing.

We look around and find a Walgreens on every corner in our area. With access to more pharmacies wouldn't that result in better health? There is an Urgent care popping up all over the place. With access to medical care wouldn't that create more health? We have massive hospitals in every major city while more and more of them are built even in smaller metropolitan areas daily. Wouldn't places with smart medical professionals closer to our homes result in better healthcare for all?

So let's look take a look at the numbers.

The Most Common Types of Chronic Pain

Defined as pain that lasts for more than 12 weeks, chronic pain may feel sharp or dull, causing a burning or aching sensation in the affected areas; steady or intermittent, coming and going without any apparent reason and can occur in nearly any part of your body which may feel different in the various affected areas according to Cirino (2017). The common types as Cirino (2017) asserts are:

- Headaches due to tension, eye strain, migraine and cluster headaches caused by the enlargement of blood vessels in the head.

- Postsurgical pain

- Post Trauma pain

- Lower back pain; slipped or bulging discs, spinal stenosis, compression fractures, soft tissue damage, spinal fractures, and structural deformities.

- Cancer pain

- Joint pain; rheumatoid arthritis, osteoarthritis, bursitis, tendinitis, and repetitive arthritis

- Neurogenic pain; Sciatica, diabetic neuropathy, carpal tunnel syndrome, and trigeminal neuralgia

- Psychogenic pain

How Many People are Affected by Chronic Pain

An estimate of the prevalence of chronic pain and high-impact chronic pain in the United States done by CDC analyzing the 2016 National Health Interview Survey (NHIS) data. An estimated 20.4% (50.0 million) of U.S. adults had chronic pain and 8.0% of U.S. adults (19.6 million) had high-impact chronic pain, with higher prevalences of both chronic pain and high-impact chronic pain reported among women, older adults, previously but not currently employed adults, adults living in poverty, adults with public health insurance, and rural residents (CDC 2018). Cvetkovska (2019) notes that chronic pain is the leading cause of long-term disability in America and 70% of those affected by chronic pain syndrome are women. She further asserts that one-half of all working Americans say they experience lower back pain every year with 8% of Americans suffering from high-impact chronic pain, it impacts the quality of life of 2 out of 5 adults and 50 million Americans are affected by the condition.The United States is undergoing difficult moments in its medical care with high healthcare insurance charges that have ceased to cater to their general wellbeing but continued to be exorbitant less useful in providing the necessary medical cover of its people. The country's healthcare system is in jeopardy due to the high spending on the prevalent chronic pains that affects 2 out of 5 adults and costs its more than 20 percent of its budget a year.

Costs of Chronic Pain

How and Why It is the most Expensive Aspect in Healthcare

Costs in Healthcare and Lost Productivity

American Pain Society (2012) notes that treatment and management of chronic pain cost the United States up to $635 billion a year which is more than the yearly costs for cancer, heart disease, and diabetes. Pain after surgery is one of the most common causes of chronic pain, coupled with medical treatments, lifestyle and other disorders. The general well-being of an individual depends on their health and these conditions, however, treatable or manageable are the main reasons why people experience pain. Guertin et al (2018), asserts that Direct health-related costs; expenditures

such as hospitalizations, drugs, physicians' fees are primarily fueled by hospitalization while indirect costs; associated with loss of life or livelihood such as absence from work, caregiver time, are fueled primarily by social benefits such as disability allowance and unemployment benefits.

Costs of People with Chronic Pain vs Non-Chronic Pain

Chronic pain management and treatment have proven to be the most expensive form of medical care due to the diversity in causes of the condition. Epstein (2019) notes that the United States spends $3 trillion of its budget on healthcare; compared to the average spending on treatment of chronic pains alone, more than 20% of the expenditure is spent up. Non-chronic medical conditions are the direct link to chronic pain which in turn increases the costs of treatment. The underlying reasons as to why chronic pain management and treatment is expensive is attributed to the inefficiencies in medical treatment which thereby lead to continued exacerbation of the condition; to avert this, **patients now resort to managing the pain rather than the disorder that caused the pain which soars the expenses attached to the treatment.**

The cost of healthcare continues to soar in the United States with insurance companies reaping more from the people. Premiums and deductibles have increased in the last two decades with employee's costs for healthcare rising more quickly than wages or overall economy-wide prices, and the working poor has been particularly hard-hit. With this rise attributed to increase in population, aging, prevalence of diseases, medical service utilization and service price and intensity (Probasco 2019); Epstein (2019) asserts that high administrative costs, high costs of drugs, defensive medicine, expensive mix of treatments, wages and work rules and branding are some of the reasons why healthcare is so expensive. Tozzi (2019) notes that patients still have to pay out of pocket costs for other essential care such as medications for chronic conditions like diabetes or high blood pressure until they meet their deductibles.

As we can see from the numbers above, "standard" medical care and the theory of pain management is not getting us where we need to be. We are spending more money both from deductibles and through insurance yet outcomes are ultimately getting worse. We have stronger drugs and more advanced surgeries yet no one is getting better. We have to start looking outside of insurance driven chemical intervention and surgical techniques to help us find a pain free life.

Waiting for a drug company or insurance company to find a solution will take time and a paradigm shift within healthcare that many of us are not willing to wait for.

We must start to look away from standard medicine. We must start to look away from insurable care.

It is time to take our health into our own hands. We must understand that we will have to pay for what is most important to us...our health.

Outside of the insurable model lies a branch of healthcare that can restore youth and stop degenerative disease in its tracks. Outside of standard medicine lies answers to some of our most crippling and life altering health problems.

CHAPTER: 4

THE OPIOID EPIDEMIC

What is an Opioid?

O ver *214 million prescriptions were reached out for opioids in 2016 alone - that's only for people in the U.S. That equates to about 66.5 prescriptions for these drugs for every 100 people who reside in the United States. It is estimated that almost 25% of people who are provided with an opioid prescription use the drug for long-term chronic pain management that is not linked to cancer. In 2016, at least 11 million people were found to abuse opioid drugs that can only be obtained through a prescription.*

Opioid prescribing rates per 100 persons in the United States		
Year	All Opioid Prescriptions (per 100 persons)	High-Dose Prescriptions (per 100 persons)
2006	72.4	11.5

2007	75.9	11.7
2008	78.2	11.8
2009	79.5	11.5
2010	81.2	11.4
2011	80.9	8.8
2012	81.3	8.3
2013	78.1	7.6
2014	75.6	7.1
2015	70.6	6.7
2016	66.5	6.1
2017	58.5	5.0

Opioids have become some of the most popular medications that are used in the treatment of pain. The active compound is known as opium and is extracted from the breadessed poppy, a plant found commonly in Europe and Asia .

Today, not all opioid drugs that are available on the market contain the natural opium that is found in the poppy plant. Many pharmaceutical companies have started to develop synthetic compounds that feature a structure that is very similar to that of the natural opium. In these cases, the drugs made will yield a similar result compared to using a drug that contains a natural opium compound.

While the drugs are generally considered effective, there is a safety profile that is often taken into consideration before a patient is prescribed a type of Opioid medication. Failure to understand these risks can lead to potential overdoses, life-threatening complications, and more. Furthermore, opioid drugs have also been shown to yield the potential to cause addiction, which brings about further concern when looking at the high prevalence of opioid use in the general population.

Apart from yielding a reduction in pain symptoms experienced by the patient, the use of opioids may also bring about a relaxed state. Taken in higher doses may also result in a "high" feeling. This is why there is a concern regarding the recreational use of these medicines.

When and who manufactured them?

The very first version of an Opioid was morphine. The development of the drug took quite a significant period of time, however. Friedrich Serturner was the very first to uncover the effectiveness of the poppy plant and successfully extract the specific compound that gave the plant these medicinal properties. Friedrich Serturner was a German pharmacist. He first discovered the properties of the poppy plant in the early years of the 1800s.

Friederich identified a specific type of opium that was part of the poppy plant during his research. It was the alkaloid that formed part of the plant that caused the compound to yield medicinal properties that caused a person to experience not only a type of "high," but also a reduction in pain in the body.

Following the discovery of this compound, the pharmacist continued his efforts to isolate this particular compound. Friederich spent quite a few years isolating the chemical in order to produce a drug.

This marked the very first time when the alkaloid was successfully extracted from the poppy plant. From this point, Friederich spent several additional years testing the compound that he was able to extract. He used stray dogs for many of his experiments. The pharmacist was the subject of many experiments as well.

Following these advancements, Alexander Wood developed the refined version of the hypodermic needle in the early 1900s. This syringe allowed for subcutaneous administration of measurable doses. During this time, morphine and opioids, in general, were considered "wonder drugs," quickly alleviating pain associated with a number of problems. The drug yielded additional effects as well - it helps to control coughing and even showed the potential to treat diarrhea.

Unfortunately, this quickly led to people discovering the "high" that was possible with the use of these drugs. In 1914, the Harrison Narcotics Tax Act was implemented, which criminalized the non-clinical use of these drugs.

What are some brand names of Opioids?

Since the initial isolation of the alkaloid from the poppy plant, a number of pharmaceutical companies have developed their own varieties of these drugs and commercialized the medicine as painkillers.

Almost four million prescriptions for morphine were given out to patients in the United States during the year 2016.

While morphine is often considered the "original" opioid, there are many alternative versions of the drug available in pharmacies and other healthcare settings today. Morphine is often sold under the brand names

Avinza and Kadian, but generic options are also available.

Hydrocodone and oxycodone are two other popular types of opioids that are widely prescribed to patients with certain conditions that are known to cause painful symptoms. A common brand name for hydrocodone is Vicodin. Oxycodone is often sold as Percocet or OxyContin.

Other types of opioids that are also relatively common, especially among prescription painkillers, include:

- Codeine

- Fentanyl (Over 2.4 million prescriptions are written each year)

- Oxymorphone (Often sold under the brand name Opana)

Do opioids cure anything? Or just temporarily cover up pain?

When it comes to looking at the use of opioids, it is crucial for patients to understand that this drug is simply a compound that is able to provide temporary relief of pain by blocking certain receptors in the human body.

The drug was not developed and has never been intended to treat any condition or to cure any type of disease. Even though often utilized as a way to help patients with cancer cope with pain, the drug acts as a bandage and covers up symptoms that the patient is experiencing. It does not provide treatment for any type of underlying condition.

Who prescribes them most?

Any licensed practitioner or specialist is able to provide a prescription for opioids when a patient presents with pain-related symptoms. In the majority of cases, it is found that opioids are often prescribed to patients by clinicians. There is also a general concern regarding the high number of prescriptions for opioid drugs reached out to patients by general practitioners. These practitioners often do not consider the addictive potential of the drugs and tend to prescribe medicine without taking a closer look at the patient's medical history. With this in mind, no care is taken to ensure a patient with a history of drug abuse is not given a product that they may become dependent on again.

Patients who have been admitted to a hospital may also be provided with a prescription for opioids by the specialist overseeing their care. In such a case, morphine is often one particularly common option, especially following events such as surgery.

It should be noted, however, that even though often prescribed, there are certain opioids, such as codeine, that can be obtained over-the-counter without the need for a prescription.

What conditions are they most often prescribed for?

Due to the fact that opioids tend to have addictive properties that can cause a patient to become dependent on the substance, it is generally not advisable for a physician or practitioner to prescribe this type of drug for a patient with chronic pain symptoms.

In the majority of cases, opioids are advised for cases where a patient presents with acute pain. A large number of specialists would only provide a prescription for opioid medication when acute pain is severe. Examples of cases where opioids may be the preferred prescription painkiller include an event following a serious injury. Many patients are also provided with opioid medication after they have undergone surgery.

When a patient has undergone surgery for a serious condition that will lead to pain being present for a number of days, a physician may prescribe opioids over a longer course. In such a case, however, the patient will often be kept in the hospital in order to ensure the medication can be effectively managed, and the specialist is able to look for signs of dependency.

How long do people need to take these drugs?

While there are cases where a patient may be provided a prescription for an opioid drug when they suffer from chronic pain, this is rare, and the patient then needs to be continuously monitored by the prescribing physician. Long-term use of the drug can be appropriate when the physician monitors the patient and the individual taking the drug closely adheres to all dosage instructions that are provided to them, but this is not a recommendation.

In most cases where a patient is prescribed an opioid, the drug will only be provided to them for a short period of time to assist in the treatment of acute pain. There are many cases where opioids will only be offered to the patient for two or three days. This is often the case with a simple surgical procedure.

In one study, 5.9% of people who underwent a minor surgery continued to use prescription opioids persistently over an extended period of time following the surgical procedure. There seems to be a 44% increase in the risk of misuse when a patient is provided a prescription refill once their first one runs out. Furthermore, the risk of abuse increases by about 20% for each week that a patient continues to use opioids to manage their pain.

The physician may advise the patient to take opioids for a longer period, sometimes over the course of multiple weeks, until their pain symptoms subside. This is, however, a case where careful monitoring is once again necessary.

Is using Opioids for long term use (over 12 weeks) effective for pain?

There are cases where medications like non-steroidal anti-inflammatory drugs and other painkillers yield ineffective results for a patient with a chronic pain condition. Arthritis and fibromyalgia are two examples of such conditions. When this occurs, the physician may turn to opioids as a last resort to see if this type of drug can yield a more effective level of pain relief in the patient.

The pain-relieving properties of the opioid tend to be stronger during the early stages of treatment. As the body starts to get used to the chemical compounds that are part of the drug, it starts to develop tolerance the opioid. Unfortunately, this also means the drug becomes less effective. goes

At this time, the drug may not be as effective for reducing pain symptoms than it was during the initial stage of treatment. The patient might need to have an increase in their dosage, but this is also where things start to become more hazardous. The higher the dose, the more of a risk there is that the patient may overdose on the opioids and experience potentially life-threatening complications.

How did pharm-companies convince doctors to start using Opioids out of the hospital setting?

When pharmaceutical companies first started to mass-produce opioid drugs like morphine, these medicines were only provided to patients in a hospital setting. Doctors were extremely wary of the addictive potential that opioids had, which led them to provide these drugs to patients who have been hospitalized primarily. At the time, patients were monitored extremely closely in order to detect any sign of addiction. When such a sign was detected, the patient is taken off the drug, and an alternative would be provided to them.

In the 1980s, a doctor.that was quite respected at the time wrote a letter that was later published in the New England Journal of Medicine. The letter was titled "Addiction rare in patients treated with narcotics." The authors mentioned in the letter included Jane Porter and Hershel Jack. These doctors were part of the Boston Collaborative Drug Surveillance Program at the Boston University Medical Center.

The fact that the doctor was reputable led to the publication becoming popular relatively quickly. The letter stated that a study was conducted on the addiction potential of opioids. In this letter, the doctor noted that opioids were given to almost 40,000 individuals, yet only four of these patients became addicted to the drug.

This information caused many doctors to consider opioids harmless and is how physicians started to provide patients with prescriptions for these drugs out of the hospital.

How do people get off of these drugs?

Since opioids cause dependency, it is critical to understand that suddenly stopping the use of the drug is likely to cause a person to suffer from a number of withdrawal symptoms. In fact, some studies have found that there are life-threatening complications that can result from opioid withdrawal syndrome, which occurs when a more serious dependency has developed.

When a person has used opioids for some time, a doctor will usually provide the individuals with details on how they need to taper off from the use of the drug. Quitting cold turkey tend to cause unpleasant side-effects that could lead to the patient turning toward opioids in order to reduce these symptoms again.

How many people die every year from this?

An estimated 34 million people use some type of opioid each and every year. In just 2016 alone, according to the World Health Organization, at least 27 million individuals throughout the world suffered from a substance abuse disorder that involved the use of opioids. When it comes to deaths - it should be noted that around 118,000 people died due to the presence of opioid use disorder. In these cases, the patients usually experienced complications due to an overdose of the drug or due to long-term effects that the chemical had in their bodies.

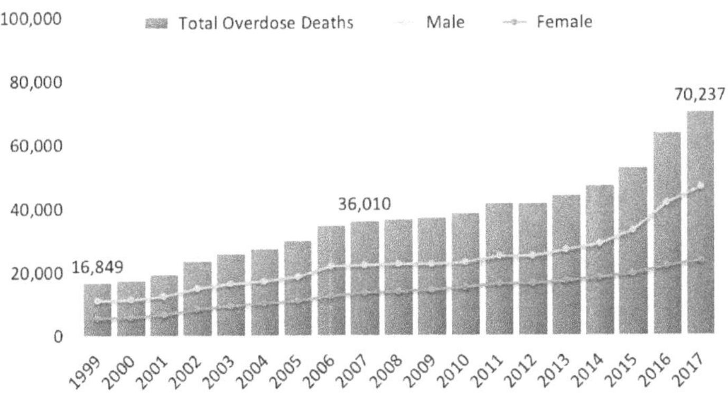

Figure 1. **National Drug Overdose Deaths**
Number Among All Ages, by Gender, 1999-2017

Studies have shown that opioids are the most common types of painkillers that cause death due to overdose and abuse. In fact, an estimated 38.2% of all deaths due to painkillers are caused by some type of opioid.

Combined with depressants and antidepressants, these prescription drugs cause more deaths than cocaine, methamphetamine, amphetamine, and heroin combined.

In one study, almost half of teenagers surveyed reported that they consider prescription drugs, such as opioids, to be a significantly safer option compared to illegal drugs that they can obtain on the streets. Up to 70%

of these teenagers also reported that the medicine cabinet at home is the main source for obtaining drugs for them.

How much money do the manufacturers and doctors make?

One of the most concerning factors about the opioid addiction epidemic is the fact that doctors and even pharmaceutical companies specializing in the manufacturing of these drugs are making a lot of money. According to a publication by Harvard School of Medicine, it was found that some doctors are making more than $25,000 just for speaking about opioids to their patients, as well as writing a specific brand name drug to patients who complain from pain symptoms.

This is an alarming concern. With pharmaceutical companies providing "bribes" to physicians all over the country (and globally), doctors prefer to provide patients with prescription drugs that they know may be addictive or even harmful. Many doctors are favoring their own profits over the well-being and safety of the patient. There are safer drug alternatives available, but these often do not provide doctors with such "rewards" when they prioritize prescriptions for such medicines.

Why are they so addictive?

The main reason why people are becoming addicted to opioids is due to the effect that the chemicals in the drug have in the human brain. When a person takes an opioid drug, there is a release of neurotransmitters known as endorphins. These neurotransmitters are usually released in scenarios where a person feels good, such as when they achieve sometime.

When the endorphins are released, pain perception is altered. This helps to reduce the feeling of pain in the body. Additionally, the person also experiences a feeling of pleasure. As the effects of the medication start to wear off, the person might start to feel like they want to take more in order for them to continue experiencing this particular effect.

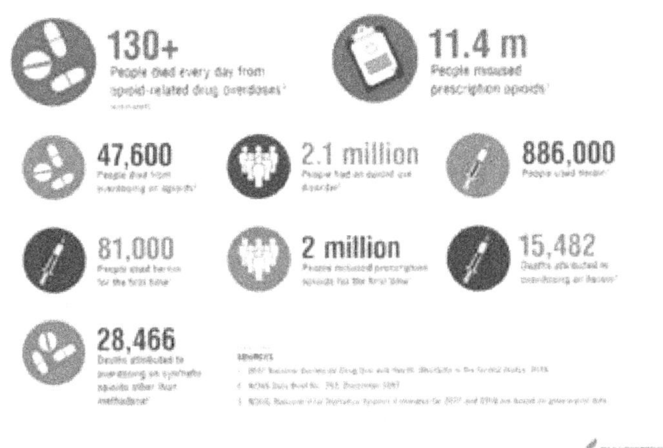

How many people in our country take them?

In the United States alone, an estimated 58 prescriptions for opioids are reached out for every 100 individuals living in the country. Over 17% of the population in this particular country had one or more prescription for opioid drugs filled in 2017. Furthermore, it has also been found that the average person would obtain more than three prescriptions for opioids during this same period.

President Trump made a declaration in 2017 that the United States is facing an opioid crisis. This is considered a public health emergency, with 2016 accounting for the most deaths caused by opioids in the history of the country - over 42,000 people in the country died from abusing or overdosing on opioids in just 2016. During the declaration, it was also announced that over two million people in the United States were reported to suffer from opioid addiction in 2016 - this included both illicit and prescription opioids.

Why does the government allow this to occur?

There are some who believes that the government might be behind the alarming rate at which deaths occur due to opioid use within the United States, and many ask why the government continues to allow this to occur. Actions clearly need to be taken, especially with such a significant amount of people turning toward the government for answers.

One common belief as to how the government is involved with the opioid crisis addresses the significant restrictions that have been placed on the prescription of these drugs. Recent changes to medical laws in the United States has caused people to find often that they are limited when it comes to obtaining opioids for the management of pain conditions.

While this move might have been made due to the high risk of addiction, it is important to take note here that people are turning to illicit sources to obtain these drugs when they are unable to receive a prescription from their physician. When a prescription is reached out, on the other hand, the patient can be monitored, and the physician is able to provide the individual with detailed instructions - this can help to reduce the risk of dependency and overdose.

Are these drugs all FDA approved?

There are a number of opioid drugs that physicians are able to prescribe to patients today. The FDA is responsible for closely regulating the approval and distribution of these drugs, and may often provide warnings and certain guidelines for physicians to follow when it comes to providing patients with prescriptions.

It is also important to note that not all drugs that are classified as opioids are FDA approved. For example, Heroin is classified as an opioid drug, yet there is no FDA approved to use for this particular drug. In fact, heroin is an exceptionally dangerous drug that has caused millions of deaths already.

OxyContin was one of the first opioids that were approved by the FDA for the prescription to the general public. Other types of opioids that also holds FDA approval include:

- Actiq (Fentanyl)

- Oxymorphone Hydrochloride (Opana ER)

- Naloxone Hydrochloride (Evzio)

- Targiniq ER

- Embeda

- Hysingla ER

- MorphaBond

- Narcan Nasal Spray

Can a doctor, teacher, truck driver, or another working person use Opioids and perform their job?

The majority of opioid drugs that are available to individuals who complain about pain to their physician tend to cause similar side-effects. The dose of the medication does, however, have an impact on how severe these side-effects would be and, of course, the risk of experiencing more serious side-effects.

When it comes to looking at whether a person can use an opioid drug and continue performing the day-to-day operations requested by their career, it is important to consider the fact that sedation, drowsiness, and a relaxed state is often some of the side-effects caused by these drugs.

If a person is provided with a prescription of opioid drugs to manage pain, it is important that they do not immediately return to work following the first dose of the medicine. This would provide them an opportunity to determine how the drug will affect them. When there is a more severe level of drowsiness and sedation, then the person should consider taking the drug after they come home from the workplace. When these side-effects occur during working hours, it can have a significant impact on the person's ability to continue with the expected performance.

What problems have arisen from this epidemic?

In the United States, as well as many other countries throughout the world, the high prevalence of opioid dependence and abuse of this particular drug class has led to a public health epidemic. The misuse of the drug is causing people to become addicted to the substance and experience a significant number of complications - and this is, in turn, costing the health care system a lot of money.

The fact that overdose statistics are also at an alarming rate is another important concern that has risen from the development of the opioid epidemic in the modern-day. Thousands of people take too high a dose of these drugs and die each year.

The opioid epidemic is not only causing millions of people to die due to abuse, as well as overdose. People are developing addiction - which requires rehabilitation for recovery. This is further causing an increase in health care costs. The high prevalence of these issues contributes to mental health problems, increasing the prevalence of depression, anxiety, mood disorders, and more.

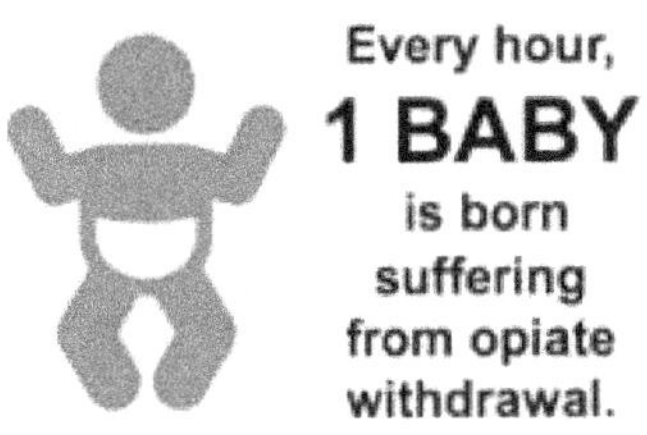

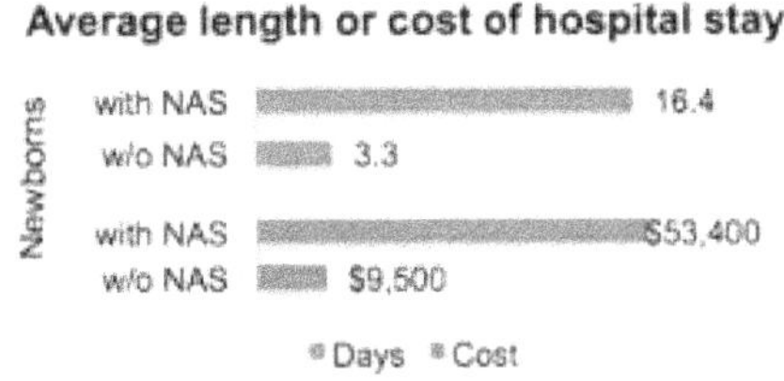

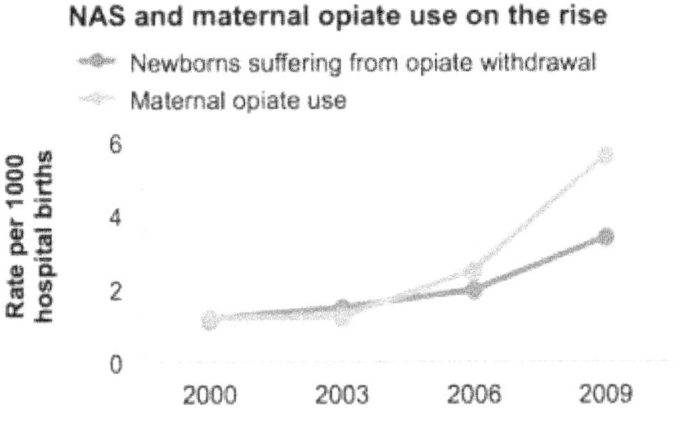

What alternative can people choose instead of opioids for the main conditions that they are intended to treat?

Even though opioids are highly effective at providing a relieve in pain symptoms, the addiction potential, as well as the risk of complications that can even become life-threatening, are considering. This causes a lot of people to seek out alternatives that would still be able to provide them with an effective way to reduce pain symptoms, without the specific problems associated with the use of opioid drugs.

Fortunately, there are certain drugs that can provide relief of pain symptoms without causing potential addiction or other issues. Some of these may include:

- Nonsteroidal anti-inflammatory drugs, such as Advil, Motrin, and Excedrin.

- Acetaminophen, such as Panadol or Tylenol.

Certain antidepressants, especially those that fall within the tricyclic class, can also bring about an effective reduction in pain. These are especially useful when combined with other pain medicines that are not opioids.

In recent years, regenerative medicine has also gained some increase in interest. This generally involves the use of adipose tissue, bone marrow, and other material that contain stem cells, in order to assist with repairing certain tissues that have become damaged - thus coining the term "regenerative." These medicines are quickly becoming a popular way of producing relief of pain but do not offer acute benefits like opioids. In cases where regenerative medicine is used, it should be looked at as a long-term solution - some non-opioid prescription drugs may still be used during the initial stages until the effects of the medicine are able to produce an improvement in the condition that is being treated.

CHAPTER: 5

STEM CELL THERAPY & CHRONIC PAIN

How Can Stem Cell Therapy Benefits Patients With Chronic Pain?

A few years back chronic diseases were considered to be incurable. People have been very much suffering due to these diseases as no treatment was available. But now with technological advancements in medical science chronic diseases are now curable with the help of this therapy. These days, this therapy for chronic pain is helping people all around the world.

In the human body, there are many joints, and people can have pain in more than one just one of them. Moreover, it can affect a person of any age group. It is a fact that these days joint pain is increasing in young people a lot due to many diversified reasons. The most common cause of joint pain in the body can be an injury to the ligaments or tendons of the affected joint. Injury may not only affect ligaments but can also cause suffering to the cartilage and bones of the joints.

The strongest symptom of inflammation and infection in the joints is the pain. Joints can be categorized into acute pain. Acute pain is the one which remains for a few seconds or little longer than this but declines as soon as healing takes place. The chronic pain varies from mild pain to severe joint pain and remains for a longer period.

Let us see how this therapy for pain works in helping people to get out of this pain. These are basically those cells which can differentiate into different types of cells of the body. They divide without any limitations. These cells are injected into the body of the patient. On reaching the targeted organ or part of the body, these cells start multiplying by the millions and millions.

These factors in the assistance of the blood vessels produce new rich blood cells. These new cells replace the old and damaged cells by healing the body or the organ form the pain. In this way, a person gets rid of chronic pain without any surgery or any other painful treatment.

Stem cell therapy is a new bio technique which has received a lot of attention of scientists all around the world. It is known to be the most effective way of treating diseases as compared to all other ways of treatment. In this therapy stem cells are injected in the body of the diseased person to heal the body.

These are basically immature cells which can be differentiated into other types of the cells and then can develop into new cells. These new cells replace the old and damaged cells in the body causing the disease. In this way, a person gets rid of the disease without any kind of surgery or any other painful treatment.

Can Stem Cell Therapy Cure Conditions With Chronic Pain?

Scientists and doctors have made tremendous advances to make tissue regeneration a reality in treating many diseases. Through regenerative medicine, a person can take advantage of their body's ability to heal itself by using healthy adult stem cells that can be found throughout the body. Laboratory and clinical research has shown that it is possible to use adult stem cells to restore lost, damaged or aging cells and effectively regenerate tissue in the body. Regenerative therapies are showing promise in the treatment of orthopedic pain.

If you have chronic back pain, it is important to be aware of all your treatment options before considering surgery. A new technique to heal structures of the back uses a component of the patient's body: stem cells.

Today, stem cells are being used to treat many types of chronic pain and degeneration, including degenerative disc disease, vertebral fracture, and ligament damage and facet joint syndrome. Research is underway to determine the efficacy of this new therapy in treating various types of back pain causes.

So, can stem cell therapy cure chronic pain? The answer is simply yes. Since the existence of life on this planet earth, people have been facing health-related issues, and medical scientists have helped people in getting rid of these health disorders. There have been several diseases which are considered to be incurable. These diseases also include chronic diseases. But with the latest advancements, even chronic diseases have now become curable. It has been made possible with the help of stem cells therapy.

In this process, stem cells are injected into the body of the person suffering from diseases. Stem cell therapy for pain could help reduce the inflammation that results in chronic pain, or it could help to heal regenerative conditions that lead to pain, such as arthritis.

These cells are the new source of curing chronic diseases like permanent cure for diabetes, cardiovascular and pulmonary diseases, spinal cord injuries, cerebral palsy, autism, organ replacement like liver and renal, dental surgery, Parkinson's disease, anti-aging, depression, baldness, cancer, retinitis, joint pain, plastic surgery etc and a list of such many diseases.

In short, it is stated that stem cells are the latest way to treat chronic diseases. It enables a person to get rid of the diseases without any kind of surgery or any other painful process. The success rate of this treatment is very good, and people can rely on it without any doubt. Also, new advances in chronic pain treatment offer hope to those who feel they've tried everything. There are many options for ending your pain, and stem cell therapy may be one of them.

What Are The Different Chronic Pain Conditions That Can Be Treated With Stem Cell Therapy?

Scientists and doctors have made tremendous advances to make tissue regeneration a reality in treating many diseases. Through regenerative medicine, a person can take advantage of their body's ability to heal itself by using healthy adult stem cells that can be found throughout the body. Stem cell therapies are showing promise in the treatment of chronic pain and other diseases.

Stem cells have the ability to improve and possibly even reverse the effects of chronic pain as a result of tissue damage. Stem cells have also been used to perform spinal fusion surgery, in which case a damaged disc is removed, and the cell mixture is placed between two vertebrae to grow into bone and fuse them. Unlike the injection procedure, this is an invasive surgical procedure. Trials are underway to test stem cells' ability to regrow damaged discs.

Also, one of the earliest uses for stem cells were bone marrow transplants, used to help patients with leukemia or sickle cell anemia heal. This treatment has been used for more than 40 years. In addition, stem cell therapy may be used to treat: Arthritis, Diabetes, Autism, Spinal cord injuries, Nerve damage, chronic pain, Lupus, Knee pain, Hip pain,

Cardiovascular disorders, Severe burns, Sports injuries, Parkinson's disease, etc.

How Can The Methods Of Stem Cell Application Affect The Results Of Treatment?

Stem cell therapy has a wide spectrum of clinical applications. But the major hurdles to the clinical application of adult stem cells are the small number of cells that can be isolated from any adult tissue with successful propagation of multipotent adult stem cells and the development of perfect "cocktails" for optimizing the proliferation of adult stem cells.

This implies that expansion of adult stem cells in culture may be the answer, although one must keep in mind that extensive cultures of human adult cells may suddenly change their intrinsic properties in vivo, rendering them unfit for restoring injured or diseased tissue in patients, depending on the methods of application.

The utilization of stem cell therapy, through the application of multiple new devices and methods, may offer rapid regeneration of effective outcome. However, in spite of the initial enthusiasm for their potential therapeutic application, SCs are associated with several burdens that can be observed in clinical practice.

Firstly, self-renewal and plasticity are properties which also characterize cancer cells and the hypothesis to lose control of transplanted SCs, preparing a fertile ground for tumor development, is a dangerous and unacceptable side effect.

Secondly, in case of allogenic SCs graft, several instances of immuno-rejection or graft versus host disease are reported, with a necessary immunosuppressive treatment to avoid immune response against the transplant and the consequent risk of infections.

Finally, to succeed in ESCs cultures, it is necessary to manipulate and to reproduce embryos for scientific use, but the Catholic World identifies this stage of the human development with birth and attributes embryos the same rights.

Thus, despite the promising results, the application of human ESCs has always been precluded by methods of application and ethical barriers.

Direct Application To The Afflicted Sites Produce Better Results Than Other Methods Of Stem Cell Application?

Stem cells in the body are tightly regulated by a host of intricate systems involving hormones and the immune system and generally are designed to adapt frequently throughout our lives to provide us with a lifetime of fresh cells.

Basically, stem cells are the immature cells which have the ability to differentiate into many different kinds of cells. Once they are injected in a body, they start inducing millions and millions of fresh, rich placenta stem cells. These factors with the help of blood vessel produce new blood cells. These new cells replace the old. Damaged and disease-causing cells in the body and thus result in the healing of the body and the person suffering from the disease. Hence this therapy gets the person rid of the disease without any kind of surgery or any other painful procedure.

These stem cells injections are now able to cure chronic diseases as well. These diseases include cardiovascular and pulmonary diseases, recovery from dental surgery, organ repair such as renal and liver, hepatitis, autism, arthritis, retinitis, spinal cord injuries, cerebral palsy, Parkinson's disease, baldness, cancer, depression, migraine headaches, plastic surgery, multiple sclerosis, etc. All these diseases were once considered to be incurable.

But now in today's world, all these diseases are curable. All thanks to stem cell therapies. But there is a dilemma that due to controversies and lack of understanding this therapy is not available in all countries around the world. Many countries still have to embrace and accept this miracle of healing.

How Many Treatments Would A Patient With Chronic Pain Need To Undergo To See Results?

Treatment of chronic pain is usually an evolving process, with medication and adjunctive therapies attempted, monitored, and adjusted as indicated by patient response. When you suffer from chronic back pain, the traditional course of treatment has been the use of medications or injections. While these methods can alleviate some of the pain, they don't always address the root of the problem, which leads to continuous back pain and potentially other medical conditions.

Chronic pain treatment is often complex and time-consuming. However, due to the nature of stem cells, it takes time to see noticeable results. You may start to experience some relief of your back pain within three weeks of the injection, as inflammation starts to decrease. As more time passes and the stem cells continue to do their job, you will notice a more significant difference in your symptoms.

For many people, it only takes one stem cell injection procedure to experience long-term back pain relief. In many cases, results last a lifetime. If you suffer from more severe conditions involving degeneration of the discs or joints, you may need additional injections.

Not everyone is a candidate for stem cell therapy, however, if chronic back pain is limiting your ability to perform your job or participate in activities you enjoy, a stem cell therapy necessary to restore your quality of life.

What Are The Various Treatment Options For Chronic

Pain

The treatments for chronic pain are as diverse as the causes. From over-the-counter and prescription drugs to mind/body techniques to acupuncture, there are a lot of approaches. But when it comes to treating chronic pain, no single technique is guaranteed to produce complete pain relief. Relief may be found by using a combination of treatment options. The following are treatment options for chronic pain

The General Options

There are a variety of options for the treatment of chronic pain. Under the general category of medications, there are both oral and topical therapies for the treatment of chronic pain. Oral medications include those that can be taken by mouth, such as nonsteroidal anti-inflammatory drugs, acetaminophen, and opioids.

Also available are medications that can be applied to the skin, whether as an ointment or cream or by a patch that is applied to the skin. Some of these patches work by being placed directly on top of the painful area where the active drug, such as lidocaine, is released. Some medications are available over-the-counter (OTC) while others may require a prescription.

Nonsteroidal Anti-inflammatory Drugs and Acetaminophen

There are many different types of nonsteroidal anti-inflammatory medications (NSAIDs), some of them (such as ibuprofen) may be obtained over-the-counter. NSAIDs can be very effective for acute muscular and bone pain as well as some types of chronic pain syndromes. When taken for an extended period or in large quantities, they may have adverse effects on the kidneys, clotting of blood, and gastrointestinal system.

Anti-depressants

Some of the older categories of antidepressants may be very helpful in controlling pain; specifically the tricyclic antidepressants. The pain relieving properties of these medications are such that they can relieve pain in doses that are lower than the doses needed to treat depression. These medications are not meant to be taken on an "as needed" basis but must be taken every day whether or not you have pain. Your physician may attempt to lessen some of the side effects, particularly sedation, by having you take these medications at night.

Anticonvulsants (Anti-seizure) Medications

These medications can be very helpful for some kinds of nerve type pain (such as burning, shooting pain). These medications also are not meant to be taken on an "as needed" basis. They should be taken every day whether or not you feel pain. Some of them may have the side effect of drowsiness which often improves with time.

Some have the side effect of weight gain. If you have kidney stones or glaucoma, be sure to tell your doctor as there are some anticonvulsants that are not recommended to be given under those conditions. The newer anticonvulsants do not need liver monitoring but required caution if given to patients with kidney disease.

Muscle Relaxants

These medications are most often used in the acute setting of muscle spasm. The most common side effect seen with these medications is drowsiness.

Opioids

When used appropriately, opioids may be very effective in controlling certain types of chronic pain. They tend to be less effective or require higher doses in nerve type pain. For pain is present all day and night, a long-acting opioid is usually recommended.

One of the most frequent side effects is constipation, which is mild may be treated by drinking lots of liquids but may need to be treated with medications. Drowsiness is another side effect which often gets better over time as you get used to the medication.

Pain Clinics

Many people suffering from chronic pain are able to gain some measure of control over it by trying many of the above treatments on their own. But for some, no matter what treatment approach they try, they still suffer from debilitating pain. For them, pain clinics -- special care centers devoted exclusively to dealing with intractable pain -- may be the answer.

Some pain clinics are associated with hospitals, and others are private; in either case, both inpatient and outpatient treatment are usually available. There are several categories of medications that are used for the treatment of chronic pain.

How Has The Use Of Different Stem Cells Affected Treatment? Is One Type More Beneficial Than Another?

Stem cells themselves do not serve any single purpose but are important for several reasons. First, with the right stimulation, many stem cells can take on the role of any type of cell, and they can regenerate damaged tissue, under the right conditions.

There are many different types of stem cells that come from different places in the body or are formed at different times in our lives. These include embryonic stem cells that exist only at the earliest stages of development and various types of tissue-specific (or adult) stem cells that appear during fetal development and remain in our bodies throughout life.

Also, all stem cells can self-renew (make copies of themselves) and differentiate (develop into more specialized cells). Beyond these two critical abilities, though, stem cells vary widely in what they can and cannot do.

In recent times, scientists are exploring the different roles tissue-specific stem cells might play in healing, with the understanding that these stem cells have specific and limited capabilities. Without manipulation in the lab, tissue-specific stem cells can only generate the other cell types found in the tissues where they live.

For example, the blood-forming (hematopoietic) stem cells found in bone marrow regenerate the cells in the blood, while neural stem cells in the brain make brain cells. A hematopoietic stem cell won't spontaneously make a brain cell and vice versa. Thus, it is unlikely that a single cell type can be used to treat a multitude of unrelated diseases involving different tissues or organs.

Scientists have learned to make certain specialized cell types through a multi-step process using pluripotent stem cells, that is embryonic stem cells or induced pluripotent stem (iPS) cells. These cells have the potential to form all the different cell types in the body and offer an exciting opportunity to develop new treatment strategies.

Embryonic stem cells and iPS cells, however, are not good candidates to be used directly as treatments, as they require careful instruction to become the specific cells needed to regenerate diseased or damaged tissue. If not properly directed, these stem cells may overgrow and cause tumors when injected into the patient.

When compared with embryonic stem cells, adult stem cells have a more limited ability to give rise to various cells of the body. Until recently, researchers thought adult stem cells could create only similar types of cells. For instance, researchers thought that stem cells residing in the bone marrow could give rise only to blood cells.

However, emerging evidence suggests that adult stem cells may be able to create various types of cells. For instance, bone marrow stem cells may be able to create bone or heart muscle cells. This research has led to early-stage clinical trials to test usefulness and safety in people. For example, adult stem cells are currently being tested in people with neurological or heart disease.

Can Direct Ozone Application To The Afflicted Sites Produce Just As Good Results As Any Other Type Of Stem Cells?

Ozone is a naturally occurring element found in our atmosphere. Ozone has different actions depending on its concentration and how it's administered. While ozone does have a direct killing effect on bacteria, funguses, protozoa, and viruses, its main mechanisms of action are by stimulating (modulating) our natural physiological immune and regenerative systems. Thus, ozone easily fits into the category of "biological therapy" or "physiological therapy."

For instance, in a regenerative system, ozone supports and accelerates the body's natural ability to heal damaged tissue and regenerate healthy tissue. Examples include ozone injections to treat damaged joints. It accomplishes this by stimulating the mitochondria of cells that are actively involved in regeneration, such as Stem Cells or the cells that generate new collagen in a damaged joint, or those that form new bones in the case of bone damage. Ozone is better at supporting the health of your mitochondria than any other known substance.

As a detox agent, ozone stimulates the body's natural ability to generate its anti-oxidants. This is particularly important for the health of the two organs that generate more oxidative activity than all other organs, namely, your liver and brain.

Ozone stimulates a powerful anti-oxidative response by our bodies and has proven effective in subduing the overproduction of inflammatory cells such as those associated with Asthma, Diabetes, as well as other painful inflammatory diseases like arthritis, Fibromyalgia, and others.

Also, ozone stimulates oxygen metabolism by empowering your red blood cells with greater cellular energy derived from glycolysis. This also increases the ability of your red blood cells to deliver a greater quantity of oxygen to your tissues. This not only increases your body's ability to regenerate new tissues, it directly attacks bacteria, which are anaerobic and are negatively affected in an oxygen-rich environment.

As the clinical evidence for the effectiveness of Ozone therapy is gaining recognition, there are now several clinics throughout the country that are having remarkable results treating chronic complex infections making it produce the same effect as other stem cells.

Are There Any Conditions That Require A Specific Type Of Stem Cells For Successful Engraftment?

In a typical stem cell transplant for cancer very high doses of chemo are used, sometimes along with radiation therapy, to try to kill all the cancer cells. This treatment also kills the stem cells in the bone marrow. Soon after treatment, stem cells are given to replace those that were destroyed. These stem cells are given into a vein, much like a blood transfusion. Over time they settle in the bone marrow and begin to grow and make healthy blood cells. This process is called engraftment.

Engraftment is when transplanted stem cells enter the blood, make their way to the bone marrow and start making new blood cells. It usually takes about 2 to 6 weeks to start seeing a steady return to normal blood cell counts. You will be in the hospital for some of this time.

During this time, you may feel tired and generally unwell. You are at risk of fever, infection, bleeding, anemia, damage to the organs and dietary problems. Most of these problems are worse when the blood count is very low, usually 2 to 3 weeks after the transplant.

In this type of transplant, your stem cells are removed, or harvested, from your blood before you get the treatment that destroys them. Your stem cells are removed from either your bone marrow or your blood and then frozen. After you get high doses of chemo and radiation, the stem cells are thawed and given back to you.

One advantage of autologous stem cell transplant is that you're getting your cells back. You don't have to worry about the new stem cells (called the engrafted cells or the "graft") attacking your body (graft-versus-host disease) or about getting a new infection from another person.

Another treatment to help kill cancer cells that might be in the returned stem cells involves giving anti-cancer drugs after transplant. The stem cells are not treated. After the transplant, the patient gets anti-cancer drugs to get rid of any cancer cells that may be in the body. This is called in vivo purging.

Blood taken from the placenta and umbilical cord of newborns is a newer source of stem cells for an allogeneic transplant. Called cord blood, this small volume of blood has a high number of stem cells that tend to multiply quickly. But there are often not enough stem cells in a unit of cord blood for large adults, so most cord blood transplants done so far have been in children and smaller adults.

CHAPTER: 6

MESENCHYMAL STEM CELLS

'Mesenchymal' refers to cells that are able to differentiate into various cell types, including chondrocytes, osteocytes, adipocytes, myocytes, and neurons.

Clinically, these proliferative cells are sourced for use in the human body through two main channels: allograft or autograft. Autograft refers to the method that employs the use of a person's own stem cell content harvested from their body (usually from bone marrow or fat tissue) for use in their body. The patient must first undergo an invasive procedure to harvest the MSCs from the bone marrow or fat. The cells are then centrifuged and possibly enzymatically extracted to isolate the MSC's for use. Although this type of procedure is usually safe, patients can be at risk of infection, bleeding, and chronic pain from this procedure.

Allograft refers to the use of mesenchymal stem cells from allograft cord tissue which is harvested from umbilical cords and used similarly to other donated tissues. Umbilical cords are preserved from healthy, full-term babies that were born via scheduled C-section. The tissue is extracted and cryopreserved in liquid nitrogen until it is deemed safe for use through rigorous testing methodologies. The safe and live tissue is then ready for use and remains frozen until minutes before use at the clinic administering the cellular product.

Are these safe?

Although things can change daily within medicine and with the FDA, bone marrow and Wharton's jelly derived MSC's are considered safe and able to be used within the orthopedic world. In addition to joint health, researchers and clinicians continue to investigate further applications and conditions where MSC's regenerative and immuno-modulatory properties can be used to help patients even more.

Which is the best? Allograft or Autograft?

Currently, in the joint pain and orthopedic arena, you will find many physicians that think their methods of isolating and utilizing MSC's are the best and most effective. This can many times be due to marketing strategy ("my method or my doctor is the best!"), difficulty of procedure (the more difficult the procedure the more effective) or just unresearched dogma (like much of medicine and its procedures based on outdated research). Some clinics will bash others for the type of practitioner delivering the care or bash methods because they may not be the same protocol as what they provide. What we must do as patients however is sift through the marketing jargon and do the research so that we can identify what type of treatment we need at what time.

Sure, it is true that belief in one's treatment method is great. The placebo effect is very real and a patient's and practitioner's belief in a procedure will ABSOLUTELY help make a procedure more effective. It is my belief that knowing the science of MSC's, however, can help reassure you as the patient what method is actually proving to be the best within the literature.

In years past, bone marrow has been considered one of the main sources for MSCs. Both experimental and clinical applications had relied heavily on bone marrow as most knowledge surrounding MSCs has been derived from bone marrow study. However, more recent research has led to the understanding that MSCs in bone marrow decrease significantly with age and isolating them can prove more work than what they're worth.

Most recently, scientists have reported success in isolating and establishing MSC cultures from umbilical cord stroma, also called Wharton's jelly. It is abundantly clear to researchers that the umbilical cord contains these all-important MSCs and Wharton's jelly is the source that appears to be far more precise and efficient than other methods at creating the MSC cultures.

Wharton's Jelly

Wharton's jelly is a gelatinous tissue within the umbilical cord that contains myofibroblast-like stromal cells. A myofibroblast is a cell that is in between a fibroblast (what provides structural framework to a cell) and a smooth muscle cell in phenotype. First discovered in 1656 by Wharton, the full potential of this material was still yet to be understood.

Wharton's jelly is classified as a connective tissue. There is some debate over the specific classification of the connective tissue. While some consider Wharton's jelly a simple connective tissue in contrast to the liquid or skeletal connective tissues, it is most commonly classified as a mucoid, or mucous connective tissue. All connective tissues share a commonality in that they comprise cells surrounded by the extracellular matrix that binds them. Of course, Wharton (the man who discovered this connective tissue in umbilical cords) knew nothing of 'cells' within his "Jelly," as cells were not described until 9 years later by Hooke in 1665.

Usually, other cells are also present in the matrix of connective tissues including some form of phagocytic cell type (like white blood cells) and also those providing vascular and nervous elements. In this respect, the

Wharton's jelly of the human cord is unique among connective tissues as it contains only mesenchymal cells that comprise the functional myofibroblasts of the tissue, and their precursors.

Wharton's jelly is gaining attention as an excellent source of mesenchymal stromal cells now being employed in clinical trials and in healthcare clinics across the world. Wharton's jelly MSC's stemness and immune properties appear to be more robustly expressed and functional than those derived from older adult tissues like bone marrow. They are considered much more proliferative, immunosuppressive, and even therapeutically active stem cells giving them an upper hand when working to heal an arthritic knee or damaged tissue.

Not only do they seem to work better, studies show that the amount of MSC's derived from Wharton's Jelly is much greater in numbers as well. Wharton's jelly has higher ratio of MSC's than bone marrow and the cells have also shown a much greater stability in vivo than bone marrow MSC's. These staggering benefits of Wharton's jelly vs autologous MSC's are why many clinicians worldwide are quickly moving away from autologous cells and utilizing the more vibrant and proliferative allogeneic source in their treatment protocols.

So why are our own stem cells not as good as the Wharton's jelly competitor?

Age.

Even though we have millions if not trillions of MSCs flowing through our body at any given time no matter what our age and these cells have remarkable self-renewal ability. There is increasing evidence that the aging process has adverse effects on stem cell viability and overall number. As stem cells age, their renewal ability deteriorates and their ability to differentiate into the various cell types is altered. This, in turn, impacts the stem cells ability to be reparative and restorative to the body's various cells.

One simple example is the healing process. The very young can heal extremely quickly from bone fracture while the same fracture in someone elderly can take significantly longer to heal. There is also a substantial amount of evidence showing that deterioration of adult stem cells in adults can become an important player in the initiation of several diseases in aging. There are several potential mechanisms that are believed to contribute to the aging-associated stem cell dysfunction including microenvironment, DNA damage and telomere shortening, mitochondrial dysfunction, and epigenetic alteration.

<u>Microenvironment</u>: Aging is characterized by common environmental conditions, such as hormonal, immunologic, and meta•bolic disorders. These three elements are considered the critical microenvironmental factors affecting stem cell functions. Changes in these microenvironmental factors in response to aging are believed to be responsible for the changes in stem cell function with aging. It has been shown that potentially underlying aging-related tissue degeneration, such as osteoporosis, could be due to impaired MSCs by surrounding micro-environmental pathologic factors

<u>DNA damage and telomere shortening</u>: Spontaneous and extrinsic mutational events happen to DNA on a daily basis. While most of the damaged DNAs are repaired by normal DNA repair mechanisms, like the stem cells discussed previously, some of the mutated DNAs appear to escape from the repair mechanism and accumulate over time. A significant accumulation of this damaged or mutated DNA may in part be responsible for the various cellular events of the aging process. Premature aging can be resulted from defects in the DNA repair and telomerase pathway components of cells.

<u>Mitochondrial dysfunction</u>: Mitochondria are the powerhouse of the cell. They are the main source of cellular adenosine triphosphate (ATP) that plays a central role in a variety of cellular processes. As such, mitochondria

produce about 90% of cellular energy. However, dysfunction of the mitochondria can cause severe issues for the cells. The aging-related free radical generation, disruption in Ca++ homeostasis, and increased cell apoptosis are three causes of mitochondria dysfunction that directly affects aging-related diseases.

<u>Epigenetic alteration</u>: Epigenetics refer to changes in gene expression (the visible results of genetic material), which are heritable through modifications without affecting the DNA sequence. It has also been defined more broadly as the dynamic regulation of gene expression by sequence-independent mechanisms, including but not limited to changes in DNA methylation and histone modifications. Stem cell fates are regulated by epigenetic modifications of DNA that establish the memory of active and silent gene states. Aberrant epigenetic regulation affects the organismal aging, age-associated dysfunction of stem cells, and predisposition to hematological cancers development. This epigenetic regulation can also activate cellular senescence, or the loss of a cell's power of division and growth. This lack of activity by stem cells will inevitably cause tissue and cellular deterioration within the body.

Obviously, aging is an unavoidable physiological consequence of living. For these reasons, continued research into the reasoning behind and processes by which stem cell deterioration occurs is paramount in the search for answers to life's most prolific killer: aging. As we find more answers to turning our aging cells into youthful ones, we will get even better results from the orthopedic uses of MSC's. We may not even need them at all ultimately since our bodies will be flooded with youthful cells ready to heal damage as soon as it occurs. We are not there yet, however, so fortunately the Wharton's jelly MSC's and other healing therapies found within the regenerative medicine world can continue to help boost the healing capabilities of our soft tissue and joints for the foreseeable future.

Conclusions

In this chapter, it was discussed what methods are being used to harvest mesenchymal stem cells and how those cells can differ depending upon where they come from. In the past, bone marrow and adipose tissue were the main ways of harvesting MSCs. However, Wharton's Jelly has proven itself to be a more promising avenue as it is far richer in viable MSC content and also does not involve invasive procedures for procuring it.

We are blessed to have these healthy vibrant cells for our use in joint care while researchers and clinicians alike determine other indications that respond favorably to mesenchymal stem cell applications. Perhaps these young MSC's can even help our aging bodies' own stem cells become more vibrant, active and proliferative. This, in turn, could help us heal from much more than joint and soft tissue pains alone.

Luckily too, our bodies always crave to be healthy so we can take some personal responsibility for getting our own stem cells working. The next two chapters will outline strategies for increasing your own personal health and help you kick start your internal stem cell activity. Healthy lifestyle and advanced interventions along with the regenerative methods we've mentioned will assist you in a life free from dangerous medical interventions that have been the norm for so many of us in the United States up till now.

CHAPTER: 7

PLATELET-RICH-PLASMA

What is platelet-rich-plasma?

The human blood is not a one-component system, it is made up of different components or constituents. Scientifically, there are three major constituents in the blood; the red blood cells also known as erythrocytes, the white blood cells also called Leukocytes and the platelets. All of these constituents are held together in one liquid medium called the blood plasma. Each of these components plays a different role in the body, the platelets are majorly involved in blood clotting but further than that, they also contain proteins that are referred to as growth factors, and these proteins are necessary for wound healing in the human body.

Platelet-rich-plasma (PRP) is simply defined as plasma that has more platelets than normal. This means that the concentration of platelets found in PRP is higher than the one that is seen in the blood. Therefore, PRP has a higher concentration of growth factors than the normal blood, and invariably it can increase the rate at which wound healing takes place in the human body.

To produce PRP, blood is obtained from a patient, and the blood components are separated. Platelets are taken out, and they undergo the process of centrifugation. This process helps to increase the concentration of the platelets. After this process is complete, the platelets are then combined with the blood that is left. This forms the platelet-rich-plasma. This is a summary of how PRP is obtained however a detailed procedure will be given later on in the article.

How does PRP work?

Platelet-rich-plasma treatment has become the "new thing" in the world of orthopedic and sport-related injury treatment. Its use has become widespread in different medical specialties, and it has been employed to aid the rapid healing of patients. Sportsmen like Tiger Woods, Chris Cathy, and Cliff Lee have in the past used this treatment, and they have all reported quick recovery, this also helped in promoting its use among athletes.

Although PRP has been around for decades, many patients do not have a clue as to how it works. They are still in the dark, and this has become some sort of mystery. PRP was earlier defined as blood plasma with a high concentration of platelets. These platelets, consist of more than 30 active protein subunits that the body uses in healing injured tissues. Platelets also secrete up to seven growth factors that help kick-start the process of wound healing. Also, platelets contain three protein types that enable cells to aggregate together and this is an important process in wound healing.

The mechanism by which PRP initiates healing is a complex one. It will involve having to explain a lot of medical jargons but basically PRP process works by initiating the same mechanisms that the body normally uses but with PRP, the process is amplified many times than normal. So PRP works by initiating the healing processes that the body would initiate, but it does so many times faster because of the increase in the concentration of platelets.

Various researches has shown that PRP is very effective in orthopedic and also for sports-related injuries. It has also been shown to be effective in many patients. But the truth is that every treatment option has its limitations. It is true that PRP can be effective in different specialties and also for different kind of patients. However, PRP does not work for everybody, various conditions like Ligament injuries, tendinopathy and ankle sprains can be managed using PRP treatment. However, some researchers say that PRP does not work for certain types of chronic injuries like over-use injury in athletes and others. Other researchers say that PRP does not work for every patient. One research documented that the symptoms of a condition got worse after PRP. This just helps to support the underlying theory that no single treatment option can work for every patient and for every situation.

What is the science behind PRP?

Some medical practitioners believe that PRP is an experimental procedure. Its three decades in the market have not been able to convince certain researchers of its effectiveness. Many articles and journals have been published over the years to show the efficacy and safety profile of PRP. Most of these articles has a lot of positive things to say while some also have some negative things to say about PRP. This section of the article will try to explain the science behind the use of PRP. Medical professionals did not just start using PRP, something led to its use and that is basically what this section will try to explain. Explaining its theory may be able to throw more light as to why its use is increasing in the midst of the criticism and skepticism.

In order to understand the science behind PRP, you will need to get basic knowledge about the phases of wound healing in the body. When there is an acute injury in the body, platelets come together at the site of the injury to form a plug, after which a fibrin clot is formed. The aggregation of these platelets to the site of injury is triggered by inflammatory stimuli from monocytes, neutrophils and lymphocytes. After this aggregation, seven growth factors are released at the site of action by the platelets to initiate the healing process. This happens within the first 15 minutes after clotting. After this phase is passed, the proliferative stage is initiated, this leads to the stimulation of fibroblasts. Fibroblasts help to create a new connective tissue called collagen and this collagen is used to replace the fibrin clot that was initially in place. While all these are going on, blood vessels undergo a process called angiogenesis in order to ensure that the injured area gets enough nutrients to aid healing. The final stages of wound healing is remodeling and scar maturation. That is basically how healing occurs in the body.

However, the process of healing is made difficult in the body when there is poor blood supply to the area that has been injured. This is because they platelets that trigger the process of healing is contained in the blood, so if there is insufficient blood flow, the process of healing will be slow or cut short altogether. There are certain areas of the body that do not have adequate blood supply, like the ligaments, tendons and joints. These areas do not enjoy the amount of blood supply that other tissues enjoy. So PRP is employed to trigger the process of healing in areas that do not have enough blood supply. Once PRP is injected into the affected area, the processes explained above will begin to happen, and the wound healing will be facilitated.

So the theory behind the use of PRP is that platelets are the components of the blood that trigger wound healing. So if this platelet component is concentrated and injected into an injury site, it will hasten the process of healing.

What does science say about PRP?

In the previous section, the scientific theory that forms the basis of use of PRP was discussed. In this section, more light will be thrown on what various researchers and scientists think about the use of PRP. There are many opinions, and all these opinions will be looked into and a balanced conclusion will be drawn.

Musculoskeletal injuries has been implicated as the common cause of long-term injuries and also physical disabilities. This form of injury has become widespread in the world of sports and this has fueled the use of PRP. The rush for PRP increased greatly when its use was accepted by prominent figures in the sports industry as earlier mentioned. According to Wellington Hsu, MD a spine surgeon at the Northwestern Memorial Hospital, PRP gained widespread attention even before science could prove its efficacy. He and his team began a research to offer evidence-based recommendation to support the use of PRP in orthopedic care.

He further stated that in the world of medicine, scientific evidence is always necessary in determining the best treatment for specific condition but for PRP, it was not the case. According to him, there is evidence that PRP helps to improve healing process in the body. But he observed that the success of the therapy was dependent on certain factors that included the method of preparation and composition of the PRP, the components of the PRP and also the location of the tissue that requires healing. At the end of his studies, it was discovered that PRP was effective in certain conditions and most of those conditions had to do with injuries in the musculoskeletal regions of the body.

Before the likes of Wellington began their research, in-vitro studies had been carried out using PRP on smaller mammals like rats. These studies showed that PRP had the ability to increase the proliferation of stem cells and fibroblasts. This was basically the studies that led to its use in humans and majorly athletes. In another study, 75 athlete patients who were diagnosed of acute muscular injuries were divided into two groups. One group received PRP treatment while the other group received a placebo. After sometime it was discovered that those receiving PRP recovered faster than those that received the placebo.

In-vitro and small scale studies have so far supported the use of PRP, however large-scale has shown that there may not be an additional benefit of PRP therapy when compared to intensive rehabilitation in sports injuries. One of such studies was carried out using 90 professional athletes that had hamstring injuries. These athletes were assigned to different groups. One of the group received PRP injections, the other group received Platelet-poor-plasma (PPP) and the last group received no injections. At the end, the study discovered that there was no benefit of receiving a single PRP injection when compared to intensive rehabilitation. This is just one out of the many studies that have said the same thing.

To summarize this section, it is important to note that PRP has been used largely to manage chronic tendinopathies such as plantar fascilitis, Achilles and the others. Some sports clinics are also using PRP to manage acute injuries. Scientifically, PRP has certain advantages and they include first the all the fact that it is natural, its ease of preparing and also its safety margin. PRP as earlier mentioned has also been reported to be active in reducing pain and facilitating healing. Also studies has shown that PRP does not work for every patient and for every condition. Overall, it is evident that the use of PRP has to undergo more research and clinical trials for its use to be fully evidence-based and scientifically proven. The next section will explain in details how PRP is gotten from blood.

What equipment is used once the blood is taken and how do you get PRP from blood.

You now have a basic knowledge of what PRP is and how it works. Scientific evidence that backs the use of PRP has also been discussed. This section will now review the principles and the methods of preparation of

PRP. Before you receive a PRP injection, there are certain precautions that need to be observed

Pre-injection precautions

1. Stop any corticosteroid medication 3 weeks before day of the procedure

2. Do not take any anticoagulant medication one week before procedure

3. Stop all NSAIDs one week before procedure

4. Consume plenty of fluids before procedure.

Preparation of PRP

The first thing to do is to draw the blood from the vein of the patient into a vial. The volume of the vial is typically between 15 to 50ml. The blood then undergoes centrifugation in a centrifuge. After that, the platelet component that has been concentrated is mixed with the remaining blood plasma and then prepared for injection. This is done by a medical doctor or technician. The injection process is straightforward. The area that is affected is cleaned properly using disinfectant. The area is then injected, after injection it is cleansed and bandaged.

PRP as earlier mentioned is prepared by a process of centrifugation. In the process of centrifugation, the force of acceleration is set in such a way that certain components of the blood are differentiated based on their specific gravity. This centrifugation is carried out twice, the first one helps to separate the platelets out from the other components. The second centrifugation is done to concentrate the platelets.

After receiving a PRP injection there are certain precautions to be observed:

1. Patients are expected to avoid straining the injured area. They need to take it easy for some time.

2. The patient must not take anti-inflammatory analgesics, other forms of analgesics should be prescribed to the patient.

3. Patient needs to apply a cold compress a number of times in a day for the next few days to prevent swelling around the injected area.

4. Patients with physically challenging jobs must not go back to work unless directed by the medical expert.

What exactly is done with extracting PRP from the body?

So far, the article has focused on the use of PRP in wound healing and also in sports injury. However, the use of PRP goes beyond these areas. This treatment has been used in a variety of fields and each of them will be highlighted in this section of the article. One of the areas where PRP has been employed is in the cosmetic sector. It has been employed as an anti-aging and skin regeneration procedure. It is commonly called the Vampire facelift. This procedure became popular because of its widespread use by many celebrities in Hollywood and also in the fashion world. It helped them to eliminate things like wrinkles and facial spots from the face. Basically it makes you face to look younger than you actually are.

As earlier mentioned, PRP is done by extracting platelets from the blood, concentrating it and injecting back to the area that needs healing. In the cosmetic world, it is also done using the same basic process, but in this case, cosmetic fillers are added to the platelets before they are mixed with the remaining plasma. After this, it is injected into various facial areas, the areas that are injected is chosen carefully that is why this process must be handled by a professional. When it is injected, it helps to hasten skin healing and regeneration. This is achieved because the PRP injection helps to increase the amount of collagen produced in the body. When collagen production is increased, new skin cells are released and these cells contain lots of growth factors. The result of this is a younger skin. The beauty of this process is that it takes just about one hour.

Is this safe for everybody?

The answer is yes, because the PRP comes from your own body, it is very difficult to have any allergic reactions. This simply means that this PRP therapy can be conducted on any patient who is willing to try it out.

This means that PRP can be used to deal with the following:

a. Dark circles around the eyes

b. Acne scarring

c. Sun damaged skin

d. Crow's feet and many more.

Apart from vampire face lifts, PRP can also be used for hair therapy and other cosmetic procedures.

What specific conditions respond well to PRP?

PRP has been discussed extensively in this article and it has been shown to be effective for many conditions but this article will close by pointing out the conditions that respond well to PRP.

JOINT PAIN: PRP can be used in joint pain. It is used both in situations where there is no imaging abnormality and also in individuals with imaging abnormality.

SPORTS INJURIES: it is effective in all types of sports injuries. It has been used extensively in all sports-related conditions. It is effective in injuries involving the hands, back, shoulder, backs, hips, knees wrists and necks. It is used in various types of injuries including sprains, strains and muscle tears. It is also effective in ligament and tendon injuries.

NECK AND LOW BACK PAIN: PRP can be used to manage spinal ligament damage and this can result in back and neck pain. There are other treatment options to manage this kind of condition but PRP is effective and also great in handling this particular condition.

AUTOMOBILE ACCIDENTS, AND OTHER INJURIES: PRP has been used to treat injuries that resulted from accidents. Accidents like automobile accidents, falls and slips and other forms of accidents. It does not matter the kind of accident it is, PRP can help to hasten the healing and reduce the pain that you will experience.

Apart from all of the conditions listed above, here are other conditions that can be treated using PRP: Osteoarthritis, Hip dysplasia, Tendinitis, Bursitis, Face regeneration, Hair therapy and Ligament strains and tears.

Conclusion

PRP has not been around for very long, it has just been here for about 30 years as earlier mentioned and its use has become popular because of its use by celebrities and also because of its expense. Because it is expensive many clinics have bought into it and it has helped them to accumulate lots of money. After the hype, scientists have tried over the years to provide scientific evidence for the use of PRP in various conditions. After much research, it was observed that PRP was in fact effective in handling some conditions and that it also had some limitations. To put it in a nutshell, PRP has come to stay and more research is being carried out to back its use.

CHAPTER: 8

INTRAVENOUS STEM CELL THERAPY

What Is Intravenous Stem Cell Therapy?

Intravenous (IV) or delivering means something through a vein. It's a simple way to gain access to the bloodstream and requires the least amount of medical skill. In fact, everyone from a medical assistant to a nurse can start an IV, so it's perhaps the most common way stem cells are delivered. Intravenous Mesenchymal Stem Cell (MSC) therapy has been shown to improve functional recovery after traumatic brain injury (TBI).

The intravenous infusion of MSCs appeared neither to result in significant acute or prolonged cerebral engraftment of cells nor to modify the recovery of the motor or cognitive function. Intravenous Stem cell therapy can promote good recovery from stroke. Several studies have demonstrated that mesenchymal stem cells (MSC) are safe and effective.

Intravenous MSC has been asserted to be advantageous because of its broad distribution, ability to handle a large-volume infusion, and ease of access. Nonetheless, questions have been raised regarding its ability to transport a critical number of cells to the area of injury. Previous studies have shown that cell infusion via the intravenous route allows a significant number of cells to reach the traumatically injured brain and to modulate significant functional recovery.

Who Discovered And Developed Intravenous Stem Cell Therapy?

Who really discovered stem cells? Is it even possible that one scientific team all by themselves discovered something so ubiquitous as stem cells? In theory "yes," but after much historical research, it was argued that no one group really discovered stem cells. Instead, the "discovery" of stem cells was an ongoing team effort over a period of many decades, and there is much credit to go around.

So, who gets the credit now according to most people now for "discovering" stem cells? Canada rightly takes pride in the work of their scientists Drs. James Till and Ernest McCulloch, who did pioneering studies in hematopoietic stem cell research. In Canada, Till and McCulloch are unambiguously called the world's discoverers of stem cells.

In fact, there were a large number of publications before Till and McCulloch's 1963 paper that presented research focused solely on stem cells and even used the phrase "stem cell" in the title. What some might say distinguishes Till and McCulloch's paper specifically from these others. In 1963, Till and McCulloch published their high impact paper on hematopoietic stem cells in Nature: Cytological demonstration of the clonal nature of spleen colonies derived from transplanted mouse marrow cells.

Also in 1956, the first successful bone marrow transplant between a related donor and recipient is performed by Dr. E Thomas in New York. The patient, who has leukemia, was given radiotherapy and then treated with healthy bone marrow from an identical twin.

When And Did Intravenous Stem Cell Therapy Start?

Stem cells have a fascinating history that has been somewhat tainted with debate and controversy. In the mid-1800s, it was discovered that cells were basically the building blocks of life and that some cells had the ability to produce other cells.

Attempts were made to fertilize mammalian eggs outside of the human body, and in the early 1900s, it was discovered that some cells had the ability to generate blood cells. In 1968, the first bone marrow transplant was performed to treat two siblings with severe combined immunodeficiency successfully.

Until recently, scientists primarily worked with two kinds of stem cells from animals and humans: embryonic stem cells and non-embryonic "somatic" or "adult" stem cells. Scientists discovered ways to derive embryonic stem cells from early mouse embryos nearly 30 years ago, in 1981.

The detailed study of the biology of mouse stem cells led to the discovery, in 1998, of a method to derive stem cells from human embryos and grow the cells in the laboratory. These cells are called human embryonic stem cells. The embryos used in these studies were created for reproductive purposes through in vitro fertilization procedures. When they were no longer needed for that purpose, they were donated for research with the informed consent of the donor.

Stem cells are the cellular putty from which all tissues of the body are made. Ever since human embryonic stem cells were first grown in the lab, researchers have dreamed of using them to repair damaged tissue or create new organs, but such medical uses have also attracted controversy. Yesterday, the potential of stem cells to revolutionize medicine got a massive boost with news of an ultra-versatile kind of stem cell from adult mouse cells using a remarkably simple method. This timeline takes you through the ups and downs of the stem cell rollercoaster.

In recent times, stem cell research has now progressed dramatically, and there are countless research studies published each year in scientific journals. Adult stem cells are already being used to treat many conditions such as heart disease and leukemia. Researchers still have a long way to go before they completely control the regulation of stem cells. The potential is overwhelmingly positive, and with continued support and research, scientists will ideally be able to harness the full power of stem cells to Treat Diseases that you or a loved one may suffer from one day.

Where Did Intravenous Stem Cell Therapy Begin?

The term "stem cell" appears in scientific literature in 1868, when German biologist Ernst Haeckel uses the phrase stem cell to describe the fertilized egg that becomes an organism, and also to describe the single-celled organism that acted as the ancestor cell to all living things in history.

Also, in 1968, doctors performed the first successful bone marrow transplant. Bone marrow contains somatic stem cells that can produce all of the different cell types that make up our blood. It is transplanted routinely to treat a variety of blood and bone marrow diseases, blood cancers, and immune disorders. More recently, stem cells from the bloodstream (called peripheral blood stem cells) and umbilical cord stem cells have been used to treat some of the same blood-based diseases.

What Types Of Conditions Does Intravenous Stem Cell Therapy Treat?

Stem cells have the remarkable potential to develop into many different cell types in the body during early life and growth. Also, in many tissues they serve as a sort of internal repair system, dividing essentially without limit to replenish other cells as long as the person or animal is still alive. When a stem cell divides, each new cell has the potential either to remain a stem cell or become another type of cell with a more specialized function, such as a muscle cell, a red blood cell, or a brain cell.

Stem cells are distinguished from other cell types by two important characteristics. First, they are unspecialized cells capable of renewing themselves through cell division, sometimes after long periods of inactivity. Second, under certain physiologic or experimental conditions, they can be induced to become tissue- or organ-specific cells with specialized functions. In some organs, such as the gut and bone marrow, stem cells regularly divide to repair and replace worn out or damaged tissues. In other organs, however, such as the pancreas and the heart, stem cells only divide under special conditions.

Given their unique regenerative abilities, stem cells offer new potentials for treating diseases such as diabetes and heart disease. However, much work remains to be done in the laboratory and the clinic to understand how to use these cells for cell-based therapies to treat disease, which is also referred to as regenerative or reparative medicine.

In a stem cell transplant, embryonic stem cells are first specialized into the necessary adult cell type. Then, those mature cells replace tissue that is damaged by disease or injury. This type of treatment could be used to replace neurons damaged by spinal cord injury, stroke, Alzheimer's disease, Parkinson's disease or other neurological problems; produce insulin that could treat people with diabetes and heart muscle cells that could repair damage after a heart attack; or replace virtually any tissue or organ that is injured or diseased.

How Is Intravenous Stem Cell Therapy Administered?

Stem cells are undifferentiated cells that are capable of renewal and repair of tissue due to their capacity for division and differentiation. Patients typically receive between 3 and 16 stem cell applications during the course of an entire treatment protocol. IV administration usually takes about 20

30 minutes. Stem cells can be administered in four ways depending on each patient's ailment and physical condition.

Intravenous (IV): The safest and simplest method for delivering the stem cell throughout the body. Anesthesia is not required, but light anesthesia can be administered if necessary.

Intramuscular (IM): The stem cells are injected directly into the muscle. Intramuscular implantation is very safe and does not require anesthesia.

Intra-articular (IA): The stem cells are injected directly into the affected joint by a licensed physician. This method is commonly used for arthritis. Intra-articular implantation is quite safe and does not require anesthesia.

Intrathecal (lumbar puncture): Intrathecal administration is ideal for neurological conditions because the stem cells are injected directly into the spinal fluid past the blood-brain barrier. This enables them to reach the spinal cord and brain.

During the lumbar puncture procedure, an experienced anesthesiologist injects the stem cells into the spinal canal through the lower vertebrae under local anesthesia. All lumbar puncture procedures are performed in a positive airflow room under sterile conditions. Once inside the spinal fluid, the stem cells can gain access to the spinal cord and into the brain.

What Is The Difference Between Intravenous Stem Cell Therapy And Localized Stem Cell Injections?

Stem cells are often essentially a type of drug and possibly permanent in your body after a transplant. Yeah, stem cells can be extremely unusual drugs, but they are often drugs even if some argue they aren't. The FDA considers them drugs in many cases. Unlike other drugs, once a patient receives a stem cell drug, it will not necessarily simply go away like other drugs because a stem cell drug consists of living cells that often behave in unpredictable ways.

What this means is if the stem cells are doing bad things your doctor has no way to stop it. You have no way to stop it. Also because stem cells are alive, they can grow inside your body, move around, and change. This can be helpful or harmful, but the big point is that it is not something that is controllable or reversible.

Systemic group MSCs accumulated early at the peri-implant mucosa, while local group MSCs were observed in various organs before later accumulation around the implant surface. PIE formation and Ln-332-positive staining at the implant interface were enhanced in the systemic group compared with the local and control groups. Furthermore, OEC adherence on implants was reduced in high-density compared with low-density MSC cocultures.

Local MSC injection was more ineffective than systemic MSC injection at enhancing PIE sealing around titanium implants. Thus, although local MSC administration has a wide range of applications, further investigations are needed to understand the exact cellular and molecular mechanisms of this approach before clinical use.

How Long Does It Take To See Results From Intravenous Stem Cell Therapy?

Stem cell therapy is the current most suitable, natural treatment module for various types of degenerative diseases. However, it is imperative to identify that stem cells are the body's natural healing elements and are being used as a therapeutic solution to fix up issues like arthritis, neurodegenerative disorders, metabolic disorders, etc. But the extent of effective treatment outcome depends upon a lot of other factors like the age of the patient, severity of the disease, for how long the patient is being suffered from the said disease, etc. Scientists are trying to explore various genetic as well as environmental links associated with therapeutic outcome of stem cells; and have been able to figure out so far that they are the most efficient cells of our body, which can produce a number of other cells, when directed through proper signaling pathways and guiding other cells to achieve specified targets.

In this regard, many patients rightfully ask the question as to how long does it take stem cell therapy to work? The evidence shows that the time required to see visible improvements in patients post stem cell therapy is variable, depending upon the internal mechanism and external support; although stem cell therapy is to be seen as a long-term solution, instead of a short-term key. Clinical studies have indicated that patients have noted signs of improvements during the interval of 3 months to 2 years! But it should be emphasized that no patient so far has reported any side effects or signs of disease progression, post stem cell therapy

Also, Intravenous delivery would have an additional advantage considering that the chronic processes leading to progressive LV dysfunction will probably never be cured by a single administration of stem cells. If true, then repeated injections over time would be necessary for a sustained therapeutic effect—a situation in which the intravenous route of administration would have a huge advantage over catheter-based delivery strategies.

Can A Healthy Person Utilize Intravenous Stem Cell Therapy For Anti-Aging Purposes?

Stem cells are pleuropotent and have the remarkable potential to develop into many different cell types in the body. Serving as a sort of repair system for the body, they can theoretically divide without limit to replenish other cells as long as the person or animal is alive. When a stem cell divides, each new cell has the potential to either remain a stem cell or become another type of cell with a more specialized function, such as a muscle cell, a red blood cell, or a brain cell. Stem cells differ from other kinds of cells in the body. All stem cells regardless of their source have three general properties:

They are unspecialized; one of the fundamental properties of a stem cell is that it does not have any tissue-specific structures that allow it to perform specialized functions.

They can give rise to specialized cell types. These unspecialized stem cells can give rise to specialized cells, including heart muscle cells, blood cells, or nerve cells.

They are capable of dividing and renewing themselves for long periods. Unlike muscle cells, blood cells, or nerve cells — which do not normally replicate themselves - stem cells may replicate many times.

A starting population of stem cells that increases for many months in the laboratory can yield millions of cells. Today, donated organs and tissues are often used to replace those that are diseased or destroyed. Unfortunately, the number of people needing a transplant far exceeds the number of organs available for transplantation. Pleuropotent stem cells offer the possibility of a renewable source of replacement cells and tissues to treat a myriad of diseases, conditions, and disabilities including Parkinson's and Alzheimer's diseases, spinal cord injury, stroke, Cerebral palsy, Battens disease, Amyotrophic lateral sclerosis, restoration of vision and other neurodegenerative diseases as well.

What Are The Costs Associated With Intravenous Stem

Cell Therapy?

Stem cell treatment is regularly in the news around the world. Stem cell providers have been able to simplify the process into an outpatient protocol at hundreds of clinics throughout the U.S. As a result; costs are lower typically from $5,000 to $12,000 depending on the specific condition, practitioner, location and treatments required.

At one time many patients traveled outside the country and were paying

$20,000 to $50,000 for treatment at stem cell clinics in Europe and Asia. But over the past five years, the cost of stem cell therapy has come down dramatically.

Some clinics have reduced prices to the $7,000-$8,000 range. Interestingly, costs for treatments outside of the US are usually far higher than in the US, charging anywhere from $20,000 all the way up to $100,000. These clinics still generally have Americans as clientele.

Are There Any Dangers Or Side Effects Associated With Intravenous Stem Cell Therapy?

Intravenous (IV) stem cell delivery for regenerative tissue therapy has been increasingly used in both experimental and clinical trials. However, there are some associated side effects. Like any medical product, even aspirin, stem cells treatments will have side effects.

Sometimes, you would think that since starting an IV is simple and low risk; this would also be the least risky way that stem cells could be delivered. However, it's likely the opposite, in that IV is one of the riskiest ways stem cells can be given to a patient.

The risk of IV stem cell use stems from three main factors. First, the cells can coagulate and stick together, potentially leading to a blot clot. Second, trying to determine the complications and side effects of this delivery route is very difficult. Third, the cells delivered this way will preferentially end up in the lungs.

What Are The Benefits Of Intravenous Stem Cell Therapy?

Stem Cell Therapy has helped patients find the revitalization they have been looking for through convenient and effective intravenous (IV) therapy. Whether they intend to decrease inflammation, aid in healing damaged tissues, or to improve their overall health, IV Stem Cell Therapy is one of the most powerful anti-aging procedures available.

With so many treatment options out there, you may be wondering what benefits choosing stem cell therapy provides. Overall, because stem cell therapy utilizes biologic material harvested directly from the patient's body, the general benefits include minimal risk, minimal recovery time and minimal worry.

The following are the most impactful benefits intravenous (IV) Stem Cell

Therapy provides, proving to be a valuable and easily-accessible resource for many health and anti-aging needs.

Stem Cells Heal Your Body: We all have stem cells naturally occurring in our bodies, but with age, this number decreases rapidly thus impacting our body's natural ability to heal and maintain optimal cellular function. By introducing a high concentration of stem cells, we are then able to heal and perform on a cellular level in ways that we have not been capable of since birth. Stem cells are so important because they have the unique ability to split in two, with one half becoming whatever type of cell our body needs while the other half remains a stem cell.

Stem Cells are a Natural Source of Resurgence: The "Fountain of

Youth" has been sought after for hundreds of years by those hoping to capture and bottle youthfulness and vitality forever. While there's no true source for immortality, stem cells aide adults in living healthier, happier lives full of activity and vigor long after their youth has passed. One of the greatest benefits of improving your health using stem cells is that they are a natural source of resurgence.

Treats Neurodegenerative Diseases: Recent progress in the treatment of diseases like Parkinson's, Huntington's, Alzheimer's and stroke recovery show that transplanted adult stem cells can be used to form new brain cells, neurons, and synapses following cognitive degeneration or brain injuries. Recent findings show that stem cells can improve synaptic circuits, optimize functional recovery, offer relief from degeneration symptoms, slow down disease progression and potentially even more.

Improving the formation of new capillaries: Although more research is needed to assess the safety and efficacy of this approach, stem cell types used in heart disease treatment include: embryonic stem (ES) cells, cardiac stem cells, myoblasts (muscle stem cells), adult bone marrow-derived cells, umbilical cord blood cells, mesenchymal cells (bone marrow-derived cells) and endothelial progenitor cells (these form the interior lining of blood vessels).

Helps Heal Wounds and Incisions: Studies have found that stem cell treatments can help improve the growth of healthy new skin tissue, improve collagen production, stimulate hair growth after loss or incisions, and help replace scar tissue with newly formed healthy tissue.

One of the ways stem cells help facilitate wound healing is by increasing collagen concentrations in the skin, which shrinks as it matures and thereby strengthens and tightens the damaged area. This same mechanism also applies to treat connective tissue injuries related to collagen/cartilage loss, such as those caused by osteoarthritis or overuses that affect ligaments or tendons.

CHAPTER: 9

THE POWER OF PEPTIDE THERAPEUTICS

Introduction

A peptide is formed by the collection of amino acids in the form of short chains. The amino acids are connected via peptide bonds to form peptides. The peptides look like proteins; however, they are shorter in length. They are considered to be short chains of two or more amino acids. In other words, the shorter versions of proteins are called peptides. Peptides can regulate the body's physiological function and provide nutrition to the body. It almost affects the body of all metabolic synthesis. Peptides may be subdivided into oligopeptides and polypeptides.

Since the invention of insulin in the 1920s, peptide therapeutics has gained prominent importance. They enter clinical development every day to treat various diseases. There are around 60 peptide drugs that have shown promising results in the treatment of diseases and are FDA approved in the United States. The peptide drugs include not only traditional focused endogenous human peptides but also the ones extracted from other natural sources as well as the ones created through medicinal chemistry efforts. There is a rich source of peptide therapeutics; they can be mined from a variety of unicellular and multicellular organisms as well as from recombinant and chemical libraries. Peptides offer a chemical diversity greater than that of any other class of biological molecules.

The peptides are used to form many cosmetic and health-related products such as medicines because of their anti-aging, anti-inflammatory effects.

They also play an important role in building muscles. This chapter explains the anti-aging and anti-inflammatory properties of peptides. Moreover, it describes how the peptides are used to destroy the cancer cells, to treat various chronic diseases, and to promote a long healthy life.

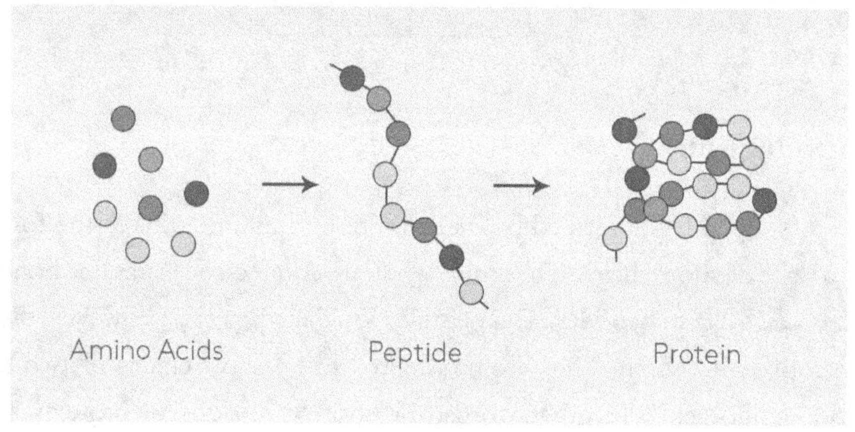

Figure 1

Image link: https://www.colorescience.com/learn/files/2018-07/amino-acids-peptide-protein.jpg

History of peptides

Secretin was discovered in 1902 by the hard work of Starling and Bayliss. In their study, they found that the acid coming from the stomach when entered jejuna mucosa, it liberated a chemical messenger which excited the pancreas to secrete pancreatic juice. It was the first peptide found naturally in the body. The discovery of secretin made advancements in endocrinology. Substance P (SP) was discovered in 1931 in the study conducted by Ulf von and John H. Gaddum. They found that the substance P induced intestinal contraction in vitro and was also a vasodilator. The neuropeptides were discovered when the peptides showed a significant effect on the nervous system. Then in 1953, a hormone called oxytocin was discovered by Vincent du Vigneaud. It is a peptide hormone that plays a role in reproduction and sexual intimacy in humans. Oxytocin was the first peptide hormone whose amino acid sequence was determined. He also produced it by artificial means. The Nerve Growth Factor (NGF) is a neuropeptide that helps in the growth, proliferation, maintenance, and survival of certain target neurons. It was discovered in 1960 by Rita Levi-Montalcini. At the end of the 1950s, Robert Bruce Merrifield invents solid-phase peptide synthesis (SPPS). In 1965, scientists from China completed the synthesis of insulin, which is the world's first synthetic peptide. The first genetically engineered, synthetic "human" insulin was produced in 1978 using E. coli bacteria to produce the insulin. Beginning in 1970, neuropeptide becomes the research hotspot. Then enkephalin and opioid peptides have been found.

Diseases treated by peptides

Peptides are receiving increasing interest as clinical therapeutics. These highly tunable molecules can be tailored to achieve desirable biocompatibility and biodegradability with simultaneously selective and potent therapeutic effects. The peptide products' vast clinical potential is reflected in the 60 plus peptide-based therapeutics already on the market, and the further 500 derivatives currently in developmental stages. Peptides are proving effective for a multitude of disease states, including:

- Type 2 diabetes (controlled using the licensed glucagon-like peptide-1 receptor liraglutide) (Garber)

- Irritable bowel syndrome managed with linaclotide (currently at approval stages) (Busby)

- Acromegaly (treated with octapeptide somatostatin analogs lanreotide and octreotide) (de Menis)

- Selective or broad-spectrum microbicidal agents such as the Gram-positive selective PTP-7 and antifungal heliomicin. (Rafferty)

- Anticancer agents, including goserelin, used as either adjuvant or monotherapy for prostate and breast cancer, and the first marketed peptide derived vaccine against prostate cancer, sipuleucel-T. (Cheer)

What are anti-aging protocols with the applications of NAD+, oxidation, and HIF-1?

The properties of Nicotinamide adenine dinucleotide (NAD +) biosynthesis has attracted a lot of interest in the field of medicine. Due to the foundational decline of NAD+, aging has prevailed. Moreover, if the function of NAD+ biosynthesis is disturbed, the pathophysiologies of different infections, including age-related metabolic issues, neurodegenerative ailments, and mental issues, are caused. The sirtuins, NAD+ subordinate proteins are engaged with the movement of such issues. According to recent researches, NAD + biosynthesis participates as a potential objective for counteracting and treating age-related problems. Therefore, the NAD+ intermediates for example, nicotinamide riboside has shown promising results as anti-aging products.

Notably, oxidation, a similar concoction response that makes iron rust, assumes a likewise destructive job in our bodies. The procedure is called oxidative stress. The oxidation of oxidative pressure step by step harms solid cells. It adds to serious disorders running from Alzheimer's, coronary illness, and stroke to macular degeneration (the main source of grown-up visual deficiency) and malignant growth. Oxidation also plays a critical role in aging. Oxidative stress happens when the body's system for killing profoundly dangerous synthetic compounds known as free radicals is overburdened. Free radicals play out some fundamental capacities inside the body; however, they can likewise take an interest in undesirable side responses that reason cell harm. (Harraan). Many types of malignant growth, for instance, are believed to be the consequence of responses between free radicals and DNA. Oxidative stress prompts a raised oxidation of macromolecules, for example, DNA, lipids, and proteins. It was proposed that age-related amassing of harmed, oxidized, and accumulated proteins may add to the maturing procedure (Hipkiss) (Höhn).

The hypoxia-inducible factor HIF-1 functions as both a positive and negative modulator of aging. In 2009, it was reported that activation of HIF-1 could increase life span in *C. elegans* by a mechanism that is genetically distinct from both dietary restriction and insulin-like signaling. (Mehta) Soon after that, work from 3 different labs confirmed the results, but also made the surprising observation that deletion of HIF-1 could also extend life span.

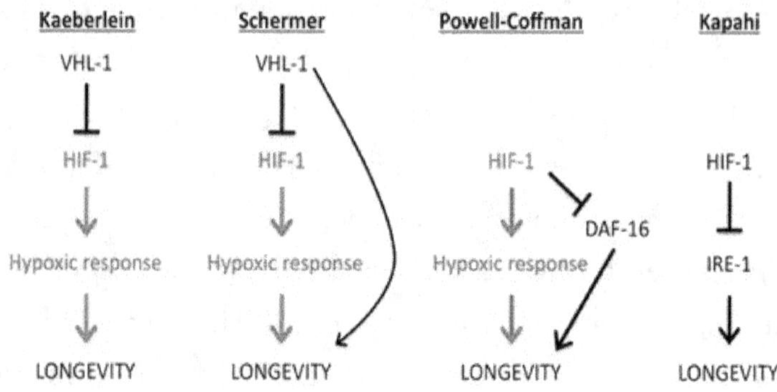

Figure 1. Models of HIF-1 in aging. In 2009, three of four groups defined the hypoxic response (red) as an important longevity-promoting pathway that is distinct from insulin-like signaling and dietary restriction. Two groups also identified a longevity-limiting role for HIF-1 (deletion increases life span), but differ on the downstream mechanism.

Figure: 2

Image link: http://www.kaeberleinlab.org/uploads/hif_model

What laboratory tests are usually ordered?

The laboratory test used to check the amount of insulin in the body is called a C-peptide test. This test checks the degree of C-peptide in your blood or urine. C-peptide is a substance made in the pancreas, alongside insulin. Insulin is a hormone that controls the body's (glucose) levels. On the off chance that your body doesn't make the perfect measure of insulin, it might be an indication of diabetes. The health practitioners use the C-peptide test to rule out diabetes.

C-peptide and insulin are discharged from the pancreas simultaneously and in about equivalent sums. So a C-peptide test can show how a lot of insulin your body is making. This test can be a decent method to quantify insulin levels since C-peptide will, in general, remain in the body longer than insulin.

What are the uses of peptides in the treatment of various chronic infections and diseases?

The therapeutic peptides are used in the treatment of many types of chronic infections and diseases because of their significant properties. They are small in size, easily penetrable, and are easy to synthesize. They also have high activity, specificity, and affinity. They have minimal drug-drug interaction and biological and chemical diversity. The peptides do not accumulate in the organs of the body, which helps in eliminating their toxic side-effect factor. Their advantages also include that they can also be rapidly synthesized, and easily modified and are less immunogenic than recombinant antibodies or proteins. Therapeutic peptides show great potential in the treatment of many diseases. In the case of cancer, these peptides can be used in a variety of ways, including carrying cytotoxic drugs, vaccines, hormones and radionuclides. The α-helical antimicrobial peptides AMPs are produced by bacteria, viruses, plants, and animals. They may be considered as a new class of drugs intended for the prophylaxis and treatment of both systemic and topical infections. Peptides, specifically α-helical antimicrobial peptides (AMPs), possess antimicrobial properties and help in treating osteomyelitis and infections caused due to implants.

(Melicherčík). Moreover, the topical application of the AMPs can be used to treat wounds and bacterial infections of the skin. (Pfalzgraff)

How does macrophage staging play a critical part in managing the immune-signaling nature of peptides?

Macrophages are professional phagocytes of the innate immune system, providing the first line of defense against infections. According to studies, macrophages play an important role in the clearance of harmful bacteria such as S. aureus in the infected mice. Antimicrobial peptides (AMPs) are important components of the innate immune defense against a wide range of invading pathogens. According to several reports, it has been demonstrated that AMPs were capable of activating macrophage function. Peptides derived from fish have shown strong immunomodulatory effects in animals that may be due to enhanced **macrophage** activity and lymphocyte proliferation, natural killer cell activity, and cytokine regulation. (Yang)

What is the role of peptides in cancer cell death?

Peptides may be utilized directly as cytotoxic agents through various mechanisms or may act as carriers of cytotoxic agents and radioisotopes by specifically targeting cancer cells. Their advantages include low intrinsic toxicity, high tissue penetration for their small size, cell diffusion and permeability. The antimicrobial peptides AMP/pore-forming peptides target cancer cell membranes and can induce cell death either by necrosis or apoptosis. In necrosis, the AMPs target the negatively-charged molecules on the cancer cell membrane, and cause cell lyses; while in apoptosis, they disrupt the mitochondrial membrane.

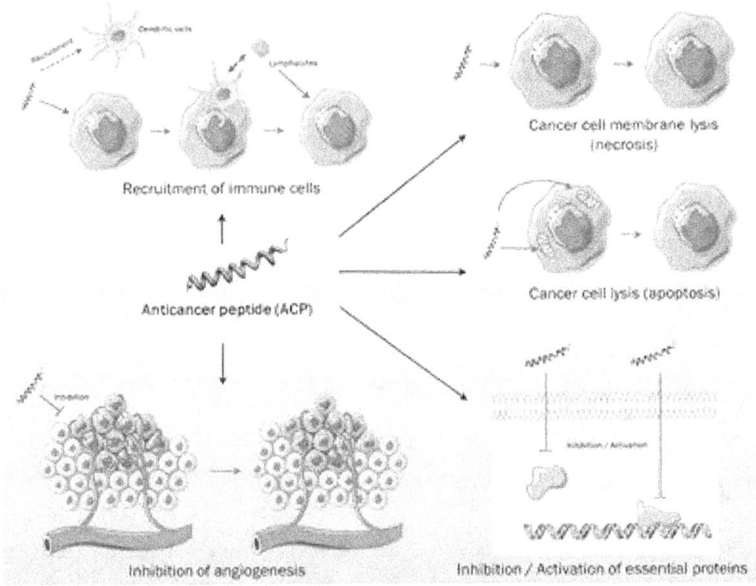

Figure 3: Peptides having dual Antimicrobial and Anti-cancer function

Image link:

*https://www.frontiersin.org/files/MyHome%20Article%20Library/248
375/248375_Thumb_400.jpg*

The potential of peptides in cancer treatment is evident from a variety of different strategies that are available to address the progression of tumor growth and propagation of the disease. The use of peptides that can directly target cancer cells without affecting normal cells (targeted therapy) is evolving as an alternative strategy to conventional chemotherapy. Peptide can be utilized directly as a cytotoxic agent through various mechanisms or can act as a carrier of cytotoxic agents and radioisotopes by specifically targeting cancer cells. Peptide-based hormonal therapy has been extensively studied and utilized for the treatment of breast and prostate cancers. Discovery of several protein/peptide receptors and tumor-related peptides and proteins is expected to create a "new wave" of more effective and selective anticancer drugs in the future, capturing the large share of the therapeutic cancer market (Enbäck).

What are appropriate and applicable nutrition and supplementation to support peptide health?

Food-derived bioactive peptides play their role in the hydrolysis of the parent protein source, forming specific amino acid sequences. These sequences exert a positive impact on the body by enhancing the physiological effects of different systems of the body even better than the effects of the individual amino acids they contain. The bioactive peptides have beneficial effects relating to optimal physical and mental health after being cleaved from the native protein by digestion, fermentation, or specific processing. They may also reduce the risk of disease. (Chakrabarti)

Bioactive peptides extracted from milk have been among the principal food-derived peptides examined. Milk is wealthy in caseins and whey proteins. Upon further processing, for example, enzymatic hydrolysis, absorption, and maturation, these two products can offer ascent to various peptides with bioactive properties. An egg is another nutritious dietary part that is a reservoir for some bioactive peptides. Fish and meat are significantly rich in dietary protein. Ongoing discoveries propose they additionally add to human wellbeing through the age of bioactive peptides. Plant-determined foods are another significant source for bioactive mixes, including numerous peptides and protein hydrolysates.

Collagen is full of useful peptides with biological activity (Fu). Collagen peptides have been appeared to display significant physiological capacities with a positive effect on the wellbeing of the body. Various examiners have indicated that collagen peptides help in the improvement of skin flexibility and elasticity (Proksch). It recuperates lost ligament tissue. (McAlindon). It helps in decreasing movement-related joint point and helps in strengthening ligaments and tendons, (Zdzieblik, "Collagen peptide supplementation in combination with resistance training improves body composition and increases muscle strength in elderly sarcopenic men: a randomised controlled trial.") It helps in building muscle mass in old men, supports premenopausal women health and expanded bone mineral thickness in postmenopausal women (Jendricke). These examinations have explored supplementation with dosages of 2.5 to 15 g of bioactive collagen peptides over time of three to year and a half. The advantages are clarified by the capacity of bioactive collagen peptides to upregulate the union of extracellular matrix proteins in different tissues by means of a stimulatory cell impact while providing the specific amino acid building blocks for body collagens.

How do peptides affect inflammation and promote longevity?

Anti-inflammatory effect of peptide:

Recent in vitro and in vivo studies have shown a potential anti-inflammatory activity of several bioactive peptides derived mostly from bovine milk, eggs, soy, and fish. The available evidence suggests that the anti-inflammatory activity of bioactive peptides is mainly due to the modulation of transcription factors, kinases (NF-kB and MAPK) and/or cytosolic compounds (IPP and VPP peptides, derived from the bacterial fermentation of casein, show anti-inflammatory activity; they prevent the formation of atherosclerotic plaque by inhibiting the pro-inflammatory JNK-MAPK pathways. Peptides derived from soy, beans, and milk have also shown anti-inflammatory effects on intestinal inflammation among their mechanisms of action, these peptides may inhibit the expression of pro-inflammatory cytokines and chemokines. (Cicero)

Peptides effect on longevity:

A person's longevity depends on their genetics (30%) and epigenetics (70%), i.e., adherence to a proper biorhythm and a healthy diet, physical exercise, timely medical care, and use of drugs, peptide bioregulators included. Peptides are signal molecules that are composed of amino acids. They regulate the activity of genes, which, in turn, control the synthesis of proteins. Epithalamion is the result of research on peptide bioregulators that was conducted by a team of scientists from the S.M. Kirov Military Medical Academy (Anisimov). It is a drug extracted from the epiphysis of calves. The use of this drug resulted in an increase of longevity by 30-40% in different models, which has become the world record. This way, scientists proved that it is possible to prolong one's life by up to 40%.

What effects do peptides have on chronic illness?

Peptides show promising results in preventing kidneys from nephritis. (Vegt) Peptides have antioxidant, antimicrobial, and antithrombotic effects. Peptides inhibitors are used in neurodegenerative diseases. (Baig) Carnosine, defensins, dermcidin, and hepcidin are the therapeutic peptides. Over the past few years, researchers have investigated different types of bioactive peptides derived from heterogeneous sources, such as fish, milk, meat and plant derivatives, which have potential antihypertensive activity. The peptides are used to control hypertension. The clinical efficacy of antihypertensive bioactive peptides depends substantially on two factors: their resistance to degradation by gastrointestinal peptidases, and their absorption into the bloodstream. The bioactive peptides with the most clinical evidence for inducing a reduction in cholesterolemia are those derived from soy, lupine, and milk proteins.

CHAPTER: 10

THE IMPORTANCE OF HORMONES

INTRODUCTION

The human body is bound together via internal networks and systems that regulate and control the body's functions. One of the most important of these systems is the Endocrine System. With the nervous system's help, the endocrine system maintains and controls the body's complex functions throughout the human life span.

However, one must wonder, "how does the endocrine system communicate with the rest of the body?" The answer is hormones. A hormone is a chemical compound produced by different cells working inside the body through the Endocrine System. The hormone is sent into the bloodstream to communicate with the different parts of your body. These hormones make sure that organs can keep functioning without any problems. This is why hormones are called the "chemical messengers" of the body. The role of the hormones is to help the body communicate internally with different organs. This way, the endocrine system can control and regulate the body's functions with the help of hormones.

This chapter will give you an overview and an insight into different types, roles, and functions of hormones and how these impact the overall health and vitality of the host. Hormones play an important role in our growth and development, digestion, reproduction, and mood. An imbalance of hormones can contribute to health issues, such as diabetes, weight problems, and obesity, etc. We will also take an in-depth and a brief look at different strategies to keep the hormones in balance and maintain their longevity with the help of routine strategies.

1. What Are the Different Types of Hormones and Their Respective Functions?

The endocrine glands produce several types of hormones, and all of those hormones have different effects on the shape of our body. Some of these hormones are produced to control the development of our bodies at an early stage. Others regulate digestion and metabolism functions.

i.   Thyroid Hormones:

There are two different variants of hormones released by thyroid glands: Triiodothyronine (T3) and Thyroxine (T4). These hormones are basically responsible for regulating and monitoring the functions of metabolism within our bodies. Since metabolism is the process of breaking down the food and distributing the nutrients across the body, these hormones also regulate weight, energy levels, temperature, etc.

ii.   Estrogen:

Ovaries produce and release this female sex hormone into the body. The core purpose of this type of hormone is to regulate female reproduction, menstruation, and menopause. When there is a higher than normal production estrogen, it can ultimately lead to breast cancer, depression, etc. A lower than normal estrogen level can cause skin thinning, lesions, etc.

iii.   Prolactin:

The pituitary gland produces this hormone right after childbirth. The main purpose of this hormone is to enable the mother to breastfeed her child and regulate the lactation process. The pituitary glands produce higher than normal prolactin during pregnancy, and these hormones also play an important role in female fertility.

iv.   Testosterone:

This is primarily a male sex hormone, which is an anabolic steroid by nature. The growth, strength, and regeneration of male muscles are regulated by testosterone. This hormone is crucial in developing male reproductive tissues, testicles, and prostate. Moreover, testosterone is also responsible for controlling and regulating the growth and development of male bones, body hair, and muscles.

v.   Serotonin:

Serotonin has been a hormone of wonderment and amazement for psychiatrists for decades now. This hormone basically boosts our mood and makes us feel good. This is why it is also known as "nature's feel-good chemical." Other purposes of this hormone are to regulate and control the functions of sleeping, learning, digestion, and alleviating stress levels. Low levels of serotonin may lead to anxiety, depression, insomnia, and a general feeling of sadness. However, higher serotonin levels can contribute to frustration, sedation, and a general feeling of confusion or loss.

2.   What Is Inflammation?

The human body is equipped with a natural set of defense mechanisms. From white cells to the immune system, the body is prepared to fight any intruders and invasive foreign bodies. Inflammation is just a biological and natural response of the body to fight against an intruder and remove it from the system.

Any invasion from outsider bacteria, viruses, or pathogens is considered a hostile act, and the body launches a biological response, inflammation, to fight the invaders. However, there are times when the body starts treating internal cells and organs as invaders, and this causes auto-immune diseases, such as Type 1 Diabetes.

3. What Are the Different Types of Inflammation?

Inflammation is categorized into two main categories: acute and chronic.

1. Acute Inflammation:

This type of inflammation is often short-term inflammation and is caused by severe injuries, illnesses, or other viral diseases. The body flares up the inflammation and tries to eliminate the invaders and treat the injuries from the inside. There are six signs of acute inflammation:

➢ The person may feel small amounts of pain when the affected area comes into contact with another physical entity. This means that you will feel pain when you touch the area. The pain may also occur continuously, depending on the injury.

➢ The affected area is also red and feels bruised. This happens because inflammation increases the supply of blood to the capillaries in the affected region to quickly heal the injury and return the body to its original shape.

➢ You may feel a loss of control, functionality of a loss of other senses. Inflammation temporarily disables such functions to focus the resources on healing the affected region.

➢ If fluid starts building up in the area, this may lead to swelling, also known as edema. This is often not a good condition and causes a lot of pain even with minor movements.

➢ Since inflammation causes the blood supply to be increased in the affected region, this may leave the area a little warm to the touch.

➢ Inflammation is also known to raise the overall body temperature leading to mild fever in the body. This heat is a result of the production of useful hormones that regulate the inflammation and heal the affected body part.

Acute inflammation may also be a silent one since there are times when the person does not feel any of the signs mentioned above. Moreover, the signs and symptoms of acute inflammation only last for less than two weeks, and quickly fade away once the injury or illness has been healed.

There are several causes of acute inflammation. This type of inflammation may be a result of:

➢ Exposure to chemicals, substances, or viruses

➢ A severe physical injury, such as a soccer injury

➢ An infection caused by viruses or pathogens

➢ Acute bronchitis

➢ Appendicitis

➢ Illnesses ending in "-itis."

➢ A cold or flu

2. <u>Chronic Inflammation:</u>

This is a relatively slower and long-lasting form of inflammation, and it can last north of six weeks. It can start even without a corresponding physical trauma and can continue to remain active in the body once the illness has been healed. Following signs and symptoms are often associated with chronic inflammation:

➢ The host constantly feels body pain, aches, and twitches, even without any respective physical injury or trauma.

➢ The person feels lethargic, lazy, and tired all the time. Even after 8 hours of sleep, the person may still feel tired and sleepy.

➢ The person may develop severe depressive and sad thoughts even without any change in the surrounding environment. Mood disorders are one of the major signs of chronic inflammation.

➢ Digestive issues, such as constipation, acid reflux, and diarrhea, are also associated with chronic inflammation.

➢ The person may get infected from time to time, and this indicates an auto-immune disease caused by long-term inflammation.

➢ The person may also lose or gain weight without any diet changes or routine.

There are several root causes of chronic inflammation. However, the following causes are often associated highly with the development of chronic inflammation in the host.

➢ When the body senses that there are foreign elements in the body that should not be there, it triggers chronic inflammation. This inflammation may last even if the element has been eliminated. This hypersensitivity is the number one cause behind chronic inflammation.

➢ The presence of a low-level but constant irritant in the surrounding environment may also trigger chronic inflammation. The body develops a natural response to constantly fight against this irritant, and develops an allergy in the form of inflammation.

➢ As with psoriasis, there are times when the body starts attacking normal and healthy cells and mistakes them as foreign elements. This can lead to Type 1 Diabetes and auto-immune diseases as well.

> When a person never fully recovers from acute inflammation, this may lead to chronic inflammation over long periods of time.

Here is a table to better understand the difference between acute and chronic inflammation.

Property	Acute Inflammation	Chronic Inflammation
Cause	Harmful bacteria, pathogens, and viruses. Injuries. Illnesses.	Overactive immune responses, hypersensitivity, unbreakable foreign elements.
Development Period	Quick	Slow

Duration	Less than two weeks	More than six weeks to even years
Final Results	Inflammation fades away after the injury has been healed	Tissue death, auto-immune diseases, tissue thickening

3. <u>What Is the Role of Hormones in Inflammation?</u>

Hormone behaviors and actions influence almost every level of the inflammatory and immunological responses. This offers the foundation for the idea that hormones serve as host response modulators against damage and trauma. However, the question still remains, "How does the endocrine system and hormones interact with inflammation?"

The first thing we need to understand is "what is inflammation?" Initially, inflammation was thought to be a low-level response to everyday injuries and foreign invasion by bacteria and viruses. Inflammation is your body's natural response to injuries. Inflammation heals the wounds, muscle tearing, and other injuries, and is considered to be beneficial for the body.

However, an imbalance in the hormones can either increase or decrease the inflammation levels. Moreover, chronic low-level inflammation is extremely harmful to the body. Let's take a look at how different hormones interact with inflammation.

i.   Testosterone:

Researchers have observed an interaction between testosterone and inflammation in clinical and scientific studies. Testosterone plays an important role in the formation of inflammation and its regulation. Studies have suggested that males who go through male menopause and face a severe decline in their testosterone production often experience a decrease in inflammation markers, such as IL-6, IL-1beta, and TNF-alpha. These inflammation markers are important in regulating the inflammation period, production, and processes in the male body. Moreover, regular production of testosterone also regulates cardiovascular health.

ii.   Cortisol:

While this hormone has been the center of negative attention for the past two decades, studies have shown that this is an important hormone in controlling, regulating, and reducing systemic inflammation in the body. This hormone not only controls the levels of inflammation but also reduce it in time to avoid any variation of chronic inflammation. This hormone works to aid us in times of stress, depression, and tension. This hormone functions by retaining our insulin in the body increased the blood pressure and reducing inflammation. Without cortisol, inflammation keeps on increasing and ultimately reaches the stage of chronic. Physicians and doctors often recommend cortisol supplements to reduce inflammation in the body.

iii.   Prolactin:

The anterior pituitary glands are responsible for the production of prolactin, and it is most commonly produced in women during pregnancy and breastfeeding. However, studies have noticed a direct correlation between elevated prolactin production and auto-immune diseases. The reason behind this is that prolactin is also responsible for sending chemical signals to the brain to increase inflammation. Increased levels of prolactin dictate higher communication between the brain and this hormone. This ends up in a higher inflammation level across the body and often results in chronic inflammation. Moreover, if left unaddressed, elevated prolactin levels also result in auto-immune diseases, such as Lupus, Rheumatoid Arthritis, and Auto-immune Thyroid disorders.

iv.   Estrogen:

Estrogen is actually a collection of different hormones, such as estradiol, estrone, and estriol. Some of these hormones perform the duties of protecting breasts and ovaries, while others regulate the production of eggs and zygotes in a female body. Females going through equine estrogen therapies or other forms of estrogen therapies have seen an increase in their inflammation markers, such as C-Reactive Protein (CRP). This offers a direct correlation between inflammation and an elevated increase in Estrogen hormones. Therefore, it was established that estrogen does impact the level of inflammation in the body, but the form must be kept in mind. Not all forms of estrogen impact the inflammation levels.

v.   Insulin:

Insulin tolerance and diabetes are linked with neurological, kidney, and brain damage to small arteries that contain blood. Insulin acts as a signal for getting sugar into the cells under normal conditions. However, scientists have observed a direct relationship between insulin levels and inflammation. A heightened level of inflammation restricts insulin from working properly, and this chronic inflammation may also lead to type 1 diabetes and other auto-immune diseases. When the inflammatory markers, such as CRP, TNF alpha, MCP-1, are present at high levels, insulin tolerance is also increased in the body. This impairs the natural biological processes of insulin, and therefore, leads to diseases. The key point here is that elevated inflammation increases insulin resistance, and insulin resistance increases inflammation. Insulin and inflammation go hand in hand.

vi.　DHEA:

While DHEA has many roles to play in the body, its main role is to offer antioxidant protection to the Low-Density Lipoproteins, or LDL. When DHEA offers protection to the LDL, a positive side effect of this is the direct impact on inflammation, and a significant reduction in inflammation levels. DHEA reduces the risk of diseases, such as atherosclerosis, by reducing the levels of inflammation inside the vessels and arteries. Moreover, the converted forms of DHEA, such as androstenediol and androstenediol, play an important role in offering an enhanced immune system and protection against several viruses.

4. <u>How to Balance Hormones and Regulate Inflammation?</u>

➢ Well, the next step in understanding the interaction between the endocrine system and inflammation is to understand how to balance hormones and regulate inflammation before it becomes chronic. Although hormonal imbalances often involve consulting with an endocrinologist or other expert, you can also balance your hormones with easy steps and practices.

➢ Get rid of the sugar. The majority of endocrinologists will suggest a reduction in the usage and consumption of sugar. Since sugar increases insulin resistance, and this increases inflammation, taking care of your sugar consumption will automatically balance your hormones and keep you away from painful and chronic inflammation.

> ➢ Take care of your anxiety and stress. We all know that elevated stress levels result in elevated production of blood sugar, and this increases insulin resistance. Since insulin goes hand in hand with inflammation, managing your stress levels with the help of diet, exercise, meditation, and yoga will have a positive impact on balancing your hormones and will keep the chronic inflammation at bay.

> ➢ Take good care of your sleep patterns. When you sleep, the immune system starts repairing the body and starts resetting everything. This also includes hormone levels. Once your body is well-rested, the hormone levels will stay balanced, and will not invite any chronic inflammation. Moreover, well-balanced hormones also help with other medical benefits, such as mood regulation, healthy digestive movements, etc.

> ➢ Stay physically fit and exercise regularly. Nearly every hormone can be positively affected by the right amount and type of exercise, including potentially balancing insulin levels. Exercise can also boost the growth hormone, which will keep you lean and energetic for decades to come. Although several experiments have looked at the effects of exercise at greater intensity for hormone levels, what really counts is what you are really doing. If you are working out regularly, your body will maintain a natural level of hormones, and keep you away from developing chronic inflammation.

> ➢ Stay away from hormone disruptors. These are those toxic chemicals that we breathe, consume, or drink every day. Bisphenol A (BPA), found in a plastic water bottle and other cans, is such a toxic chemical that can easily disrupt the natural production of hormones in the body. When hormones are disrupted, the body sends out a signal to develop inflammation to fight against it. In to get rid of these toxic elements, you can either seek out a

healthcare professional or detoxify your body and consume natural fruits, vegetables, and edibles without any additives and chemicals.

➢ Moreover, doctors can also employ hormone therapy to increase the declining ratio of hormones in your body. Doctors measure the hormone levels and suggest the appropriate hormone therapy to regulate the production of hormones and avoid inflammation. There may be potential side effects to this, but with the help of a medical professional, you can manage to address any chances of hormonal imbalance or chronic inflammation in a proven way.

➢ Reduce the usage of caffeine in your everyday life. Excess caffeine slowly raises your cortisol levels and slows your thyroid down. Plus, it exacerbates acid reflux and digestive disorders. Avoid any afternoon intake of caffeine as it may interfere with your circadian rhythm and put you in the danger of chronic inflammation.

CHAPTER: 11

HORMONE REPLACEMENT THERAPY

Introduction

Hormone replacement therapy (HRT) is the use of medications containing female hormones to replace the ones the body no longer makes after menopause. As the time of menopause approaches in females, hormonal disturbances are raised. HRT replaces the declining levels of hormones and helps relieve the symptoms such as hot flashes, reduced sex drive, night sweats, vaginal dryness and mood swings etc. These symptoms are very unpleasant and HRT offers great relief in such conditions. Hormone replacement therapy prevents osteoporosis in women after the menopause. Moreover, it helps in balancing the levels of estrogens and progesterone **(Limouzin-Lamothe)**.

Hormonal replacement therapy is part of broader group of hormone therapy. Hormone therapy is the use of hormones for medical treatment. Hormone replacement therapy is beneficial in males who suffer from prostate cancer or hypogonadism. Hypogonadism is a condition in which the body produces less testosterone which is responsible for the development of male gonads, facial hair and muscularity in males **(Wang)**.

In this chapter, we will discuss hormone replacement therapy, the effectiveness of testosterone therapy, prostate health, and the impact of hormones on longevity.

What are the common Men's and women's health issues?

Men's Health Issues	Women's Health Issues
Like most females, many men also experience hormonal imbalance throughout their lifetimes. The hormonal problems take place in men either because of puberty or aging. The men's endocrine cycles are different than women so they experience different hormonal issues. The medical conditions that are involved in hormonal imbalances in men incorporate hypogonadism (low levels of testosterone produced by the testes) or prostate cancer. The men facing hormonal imbalances are presented with the following symptoms: • reduced body hair growth • Low Sperm count • Reduced sex drive	Women face hormonal imbalances naturally in their lives. The hormonal problems take place in women when they hit puberty, when they start having menstruation cycles, during pregnancy and breastfeeding, and then at the stages of menopause (peri-menopause, menopause, post-menopause) The endocrine systems in women vary as compared to men, therefore, their hormonal problems are different than the men. The medical conditions which play role in disturbing the hormonal balances in a female's body include polycystic ovary syndrome (PCOS), early menopause, utilization of contraceptives for birth control, Ovarian

<ul><li>overdevelopment of breast tissue</li><li>breast tenderness</li><li>osteoporosis</li><li>Erectile dysfunction</li></ul>	cancer and primary ovarian insufficiency (POI). Symptoms of hormonal imbalances in women include: <ul><li>heavy, irregular, or painful periods</li><li>osteoporosis (weak, brittle bones)</li><li>hot flashes and night sweats</li><li>vaginal dryness</li><li>breast tenderness</li><li>indigestion</li><li>constipation and diarrhea</li><li>acne during or just before menstruation</li><li>uterine bleeding not associated with menstruation</li><li>increased hair growth on the face, neck, chest, or back</li><li>infertility</li><li>weight gain</li></ul>

	<ul><li>thinning hair or hair loss</li><li>skin tags or abnormal growths</li><li>deepening of the voice</li></ul>

When is it safe to use testosterone therapy?

It is safe to use testosterone therapy in men having primary or secondary hypogonadism, patients with human immunodeficiency virus (HIV), or acquired immunodeficiency syndrome. It is safe to use HRT in males facing muscle atrophy, depression, fatigue and low T count in the blood. However, testosterone therapy raises the level of red blood cell count (Jones Jr). Therefore, a physical exam and physician consultation is a must prior to using testosterone therapy.

It is safe to use testosterone in female having poor sexual functioning in postmenopausal women and for the prevention of osteoporosis (Yood).

What is testosterone relationship to prostate cancer, and male sexuality?

In the early 1940s, researchers Charles Brenton Huggins and Clarence Hodges discovered that when men's testosterone production dropped, their prostate cancer stopped growing. The researchers also found that giving testosterone to men with prostate cancer made their cancer grow. They concluded that testosterone promotes prostate cancer growth (Morgentaler).

As further evidence, one of the main treatments for prostate cancer —

<u>hormone therapy</u> — slows cancer growth by lowering testosterone levels in the body. The fact that testosterone is involved in providing fuel to prostate cancer growth, many doctors have started avoiding prescribing testosterone therapy for men having a history of prostate cancer (Morgentaler).

Some men maintain sexual desire at relatively low testosterone levels. For other men, libido may lag even with normal testosterone levels. Low testosterone is one of the possible causes of low libido, however. If testosterone is lowered far enough, virtually all men will experience some decline in sex drive.

What are common sexual, reproductive, and hormonal health issues for men and women?

The endocrine system plays a critical role in human reproduction and sexuality (MacLusky). In men, the testes (testicles) produce testosterone, a hormone that brings about the physical changes that transform a boy into an adult male. Throughout life, testosterone helps maintain muscle and bone mass, sperm production, and sex drive. Women's ovaries produce estrogen and progesterone, hormones responsible for female development and maintaining pregnancy.

Sexual, reproductive, and hormonal issues in Men

<u>Important reproductive health issues in men include</u>

- Prostate concerns, including enlarged prostate and prostate cancer

- Male hypogonadism—effects (symptoms) of low testosterone and consistently lower than normal levels of testosterone in the blood

- Male infertility—inability to produce sperm adequate for reproduction

<u>Sexual dysfunction</u>

- Erectile dysfunction—inability to get or keep an erection from enough for sexual intercourse

- Decreased libido—reduced sexual desire or interest<u>Hormonal Issues</u>

Gynecomastia is breast enlargement in boys or men due to a benign (non-cancerous) increase in breast tissue. This condition results from an imbalance between the hormones testosterone and estrogen (Sansone).

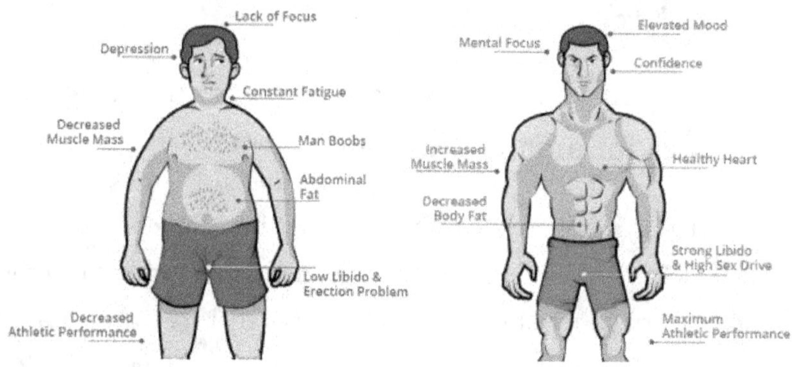

Figure 1

Image link: https://www.dailymoss.com/wp-content/uploads/2019/11/hrt-treatments-for-male- amp-females-hormone-replacement-therapy-symptoms-amp-ben-5dc430ca5a0c7.png

Sexual, reproductive, and hormonal issues in Women

The sexual problems reported by women commonly consist of three types:

- Lack of sexual desire: Lack of interest in sex, or desire for sex, is a common problem in both men and women, but especially in women. Lack of desire stops the sexual response cycle before it starts. Lack of desire is temporary in some people and an ongoing problem in others.

- Difficulties becoming sexually aroused or achieving orgasm:

- Inability to become sexually aroused is sometimes related to lack of desire. In other cases, the woman feels sexual desire but cannot become aroused. Orgasm may be delayed or not occur at all (anorgasmia). This can be very distressing for a woman who feels desire and becomes aroused. It can create a vicious cycle in which the woman loses interest in sex because she does not have an orgasm. It has been estimated that 7% to 10% of women suffer from some sort of orgasmic disorder.

- Pain during intercourse: Pain during intercourse (dyspareunia) is not uncommon. Like other sexual problems, it can cause a woman to lose interest in sex (Bachmann).

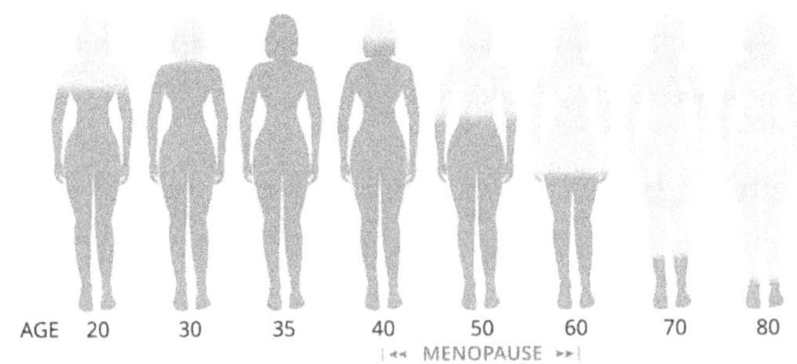

Figure 2

Image link: https://z7g7q5i8.stackpathcdn.com/wp-content/uploads/2019/08/20190829-Menopause-2_opt-1000x600.jpg

<u>Gynecologic problems in females</u>

A number of pelvic disorders can cause pain in intercourse and thus decrease satisfaction.

- **Vaginal dryness**: The most common reason for this in younger women is insufficient stimulation. In older women, the decrease in estrogen that occurs in perimenopause or menopause is the cause of vaginal dryness. Poor lubrication can also be linked to hormone imbalances and other illnesses and to certain medications. It can inhibit arousal or make intercourse uncomfortable.

- **Vaginismus:** This is a painful spasm of the muscles surrounding the vaginal opening that causes the vaginal opening to "tighten." It can prevent penetration or make penetration extremely painful. Vaginismus can be caused by injuries or scars from surgery, abuse, or childbirth, by infection, or by irritation from douches, spermicides, or condoms. It can also be caused by fear (Graziottin).

- **Sexually transmitted diseases:** Gonorrhea, herpes, genital warts, chlamydia, and syphilis are infectious diseases spread by sexual contact. They can cause changes in the genitals that make sex uncomfortable or even painful.

- **Vaginitis:** Inflammation and irritation of vaginal tissues due to infection or other causes can make intercourse uncomfortable or painful.

- **Endometriosis,** pelvic mass, ovarian cyst, surgical scars: Any of these can cause an obstruction or anatomical changes that prevent intercourse or make it difficult or painful.

- **Pelvic inflammatory disease**: This is an infection of the vagina that moves up into the cervix, uterus, and ovaries. It can be very painful on its own and make intercourse extremely painful.

- Nerve damage after surgery: Unavoidable cutting of small nerves during pelvic surgery (such as hysterectomy) may decrease sensation and response

Common Reproductive Health Concerns for Women

- Endometriosis.

- Uterine Fibroids.

- Gynecologic Cancer.

- HIV/AIDS.

- Interstitial Cystitis.

- Polycystic Ovary Syndrome (PCOS)

- Sexually Transmitted Diseases (STDs)

What are medical and nutrition products that can assist in prostate health?

Eat a mostly plant-based diet. Increase the number of fruits and vegetables in your diet, especially cooked tomatoes and cruciferous vegetables like broccoli and cauliflower, which may be protective. Cut back on red meat and full-fat dairy products like cheese and whole milk. Men who eat a lot of saturated fat have an increased risk of prostate cancer (Bourke). Add fish to your weekly meals. The healthy omega-3 fatty acids found in fish like salmon and tuna have been linked to a reduced risk for prostate cancer (Fradet). Avoid smoking which can lead to a number of cancers including prostate cancer.

Research has shown that men who consume a lot of milk are more likely to develop prostate cancer than men who don't eat calcium-heavy diets (Qin). An older study published in 1998 found evidence that men who drank more than two glasses of milk a day were at higher risk of advanced prostate cancer than men who did not consume that much milk. Whole milk seems to cause the highest increase in risk, although studies have also found a greater risk associated with low-fat milk.

Researchers have suggested the strong associations between milk intake and prostate cancer could be due to milk's fat, calcium, and hormone levels. Other theories suggest the link could be caused by:

- the negative impact high-calcium foods have on vitamin D balance

- the increase in serum insulin-like growth factor I (IGF-I) concentrations caused by dairy

- the effect of dairy on testosterone levels

How is stress management important to sexual dysfunction?

Sexual dysfunction can be a result of a psychological problem. These include work-related stress and anxiety, concern about sexual performance, marital or relationship problems, depression, feelings of guilt, or the effects of past sexual trauma. Mental health conditions like stress and anxiety can also affect how your brain signals your body's physical response. In the case of an erection, stress and anxiety can interrupt how your brain sends messages to the penis to allow extra blood flow (Kalaitzidou).

The reasons for Erectile Dysfunction vary per age group, but generally follow:

- Psychological ED (mainly nervousness and anxiety) affects about 90 percent of teenagers and young men. These events are fairly short-lived.

- Personal and professional stress, such as relationship trouble, is the main reason for ED in middle-aged men.

- Physical impotence is the most common cause for older men, but the loss of a partner and loneliness can also cause psychological stress.

- Following are some of the stress management which is important for sexual dysfunction:

- **Counseling**: You'll work with a therapist to identify and address major stress or anxiety factors so you can manage them.

- **Psychodynamic therapy**: This usually involves addressing a subconscious conflict to help find the root cause of your ED.

- **Sex therapy**: This therapy focuses on sensational pleasure rather than arousal and sexual activity. It aims to reduce the stress factor by building a more secure and reliable sex life.

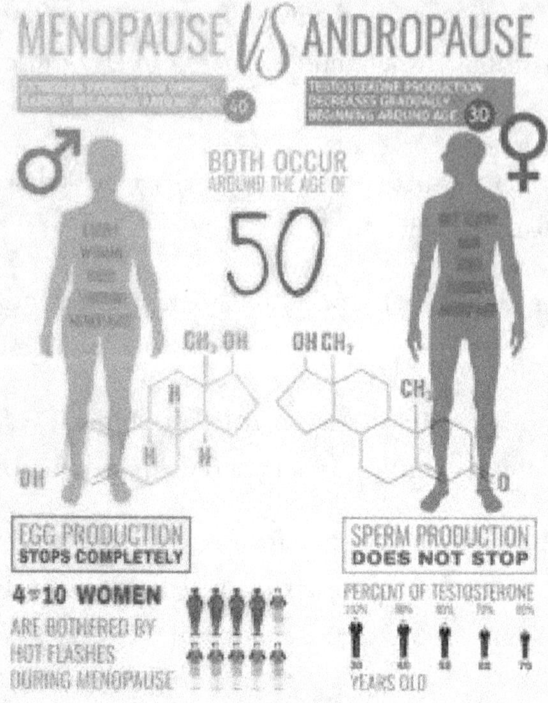

Figure 3

Image link: https://externalaffairs.ca/wp-content/uploads/2019/09/what-are-hormones-242x300.jpg

How do hormonal deficiencies affect cardiovascular health?

Long-term hormone replacement therapy used to be routinely prescribed for postmenopausal women to relieve hot flashes and other menopause symptoms. Hormone replacement therapy was also thought to reduce the risk of heart disease. Before menopause, women have a lower risk of heart disease than men do. But as women age, and their estrogen levels decline after menopause, their risk of heart disease increases. In the 1980s and 1990s, experts advised older women to take estrogen and other hormones to keep their hearts healthy. However, hormone replacement therapy —

or menopause hormone therapy, as it's now called — has had mixed results. Many of the hoped-for benefits failed to materialize for large numbers of women. The largest randomized, controlled trial to date actually found a small increase in heart disease in postmenopausal women using combined (both estrogen and progestin) hormone therapy. For women in this study using estrogen alone, there was no increased risk of heart disease.

In men, T levels begin to decrease after age 40, and this decrease has been associated with an increase in all-cause mortality and cardiovascular (CV) risk (Goodale). Low T levels in men may increase their risk of developing coronary artery disease (CAD), metabolic syndrome, and type 2 diabetes.

Testosterone hormone therapy may increase your <u>cholesterol levels</u> (Zmuda). Increased cholesterol buildup in the arteries supplying blood to your heart can lead to a heart attack. Other side effects include oily skin, fluid retention, and a decrease in the size of your testicles.

What role does obesity play in hormone deficiencies?

Overweight or obesity occurs when, over time, the body takes in more calories than it burns. However, some people do gain weight more easily than others. Another possible cause of obesity is a hormone imbalance, as in hypothyroidism (underactive thyroid gland) or Cushing's syndrome. The hormones leptin and insulin, sex hormones and growth hormone influence our appetite, metabolism (the rate at which our body burns kilojoules for energy), and body fat distribution. People who are obese have levels of these hormones that encourage abnormal metabolism and the accumulation of body fat (Rivlin).

Insulin, a hormone produced by the pancreas, is important for the regulation of carbohydrates and the metabolism of fat (Saltiel). Insulin stimulates glucose (sugar) uptake from the blood in tissues such as muscles, the liver and fat. This is an important process to make sure that energy is available for everyday functioning and to maintain normal levels of circulating glucose.

In a person who is obese, insulin signals are sometimes lost and tissues are no longer able to control glucose levels. This can lead to the development of type II diabetes and metabolic syndrome.

What regenerative and aesthetic procedures exist for men and women?

Regenerative medicine and tissue engineering technologies offer the possibility to create laboratory-grown tissues to restore or establish normal organ function.

The science of male reproductive function and dysfunction has experienced significant progress in recent years, regenerative medicine has opened new avenues for treating patients with severe andrology disorders, such as congenital abnormalities, cancer, trauma, infection, inflammation, and iatrogenic injuries. Advances have taken place in the use of cell, tissue, and organ-based regenerative medicine strategies for clinical application in male reproductive system disorders (Geijsen).

The reproductive system has a central role in women's health. Conditions such as congenital malformations and acquired pathological diseases can negatively affect reproductive organs function and interfere with a woman's quality of life. Despite advancements in reproductive medicine and reconstructive surgery, there is an increased demand for the development of immunocompatible biological tissue substitutes when native healthy tissue is lacking.

How can hormone therapies correct imbalances in both men and women?

Hormone Therapy for Men:

In the case of hypogonadism in men, testosterone therapy is administered. Types of hormone therapy for men

For testosterone therapy, several options are available. These include:

- Intramuscular testosterone injections: Your doctor will inject these into the muscles of your buttocks every two to three weeks.

- Testosterone patches: You apply these each day to your back, arms, buttocks, or abdomen. Be sure to rotate the application sites.

- Topical testosterone gel: You apply this each day to your shoulders, arms, or abdomen.

<u>Hormone Therapy for women:</u>

Estrogen therapy is given to the females who have had a recent hysterectomy (removal of uterus) or oophorectomy (removal of the uterus and ovaries), and menopause (BERMAN).

For estrogen therapy, several options are available which include:

Estrogen pill — Pills are the most common treatment for menopausal symptoms. Among the many forms of pills available are conjugated estrogens (Cenestin, Estrace, Estratab, Femtrace, Ogen, and Premarin) or estrogens-bazedoxifene.

Estrogen patch — the patch is worn on the skin of your abdomen. Depending on the dose, some patches are replaced every few days, while others can be worn for a week. Examples are Alora, Climara, Estraderm, and Vivelle-Dot.

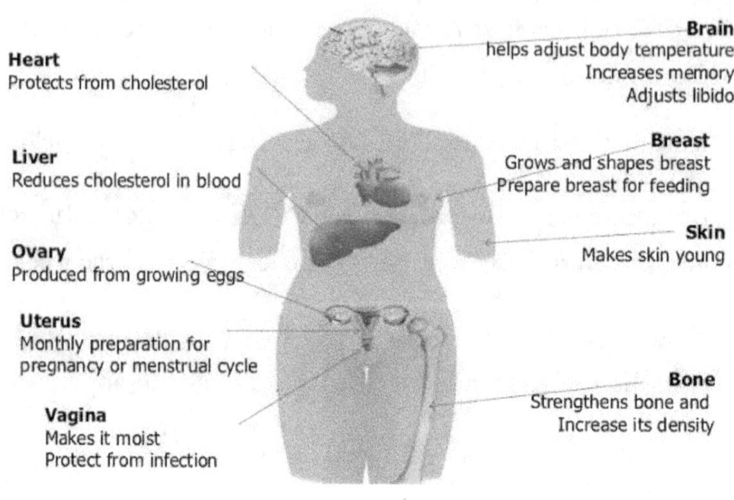

Figure 4

Image link:

https://www.troab.com/postImages/2018/5/estrogen_levels_20180515094040.jpg

How does hormone balancing effect longevity?

Hormone balancing therapies promote longevity. Women on hormone replacement therapy are likely to live longer, according to new research. And those using HRT to relieve the symptoms of the menopause were also less likely to have potentially fatal blocked arteries.

The study showed lower levels of atherosclerosis - plaque build-up in the arteries - in women on HRT compared to women not using hormone therapy (Grady).

The new study bolsters evidence that the therapy, which involves oestrogen supplements often accompanied by progesterone or similar hormones, may help improve heart health and overall survival in some women.

Oestrogen is thought to protect the heart because it lowers cholesterol and increases the flexibility of blood vessels, allowing them to accommodate blood flow.

CHAPTER: 12

JOINT PAINS AND THE INJURIES THAT PLAGUE US

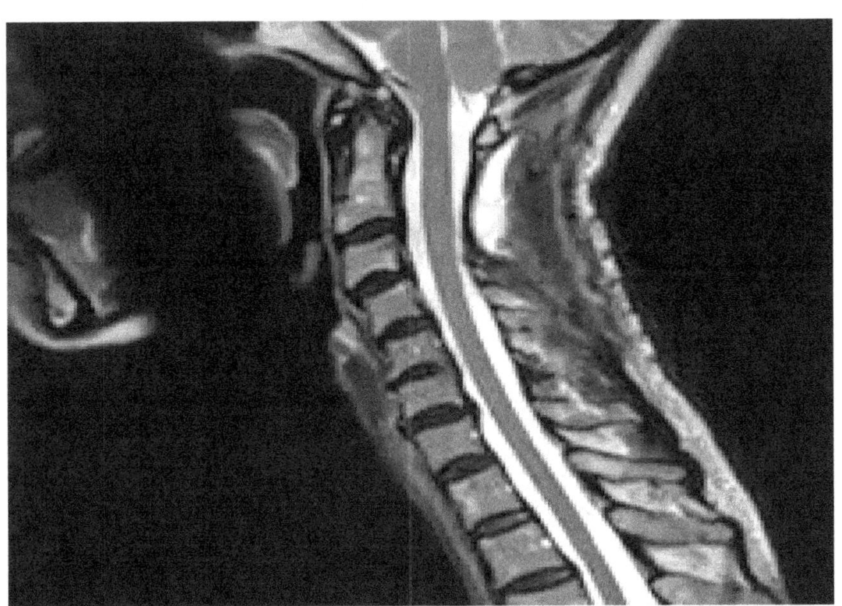

SPINAL PAIN

A person can develop spinal pain as a result of injuries from medical conditions, or as an aftermath of some activities. Although, spinal pain can occur in people of all age groups for different reasons, it is commoner in older people. As a person grows older, there's tendency for him to develop back pain, especially at the lower back. This may be due to factors like previous occupation or degenerative disk disease.

Disc Herniation

Disc herniation refers to a problem with the discs in between the vertebrae. There are two parts to a spinal disk. There's the soft and gelatinous inner part and the tough outer ring. When there's an injury, the inner disc can protrude through the outer ring. This disc is called protruded, herniated, or slipped disc, and this can cause great pain.

The treatment may vary depending on the level of pain being experienced. Many people undergo exercise programs to strengthen the back and muscles around it while taking over-the-counter pain relievers. Doctors may also prescribe nerve pain medication, narcotics, and muscle relaxers.

These treatment might not heal the pain if it is severe and the person might have to undergo surgery if the symptoms persist after 6weeks of treatment. The surgeon may either remove the protruding part of the disc and not the whole, or replace the whole with an artificial one, or remove the whole and fuse the vertebrae together.

Facet Pain

The facet joint keeps the vertebrae together, giving room for some movements in the spine. Facet pain occurs when these joints start to worn out or degenerate. As the cartilage and fluid in the joint become thinner, the bones may rub together and not move properly. This causes pain, stiffness, and swelling.

The treatment focuses on keeping the patient active and relieving the pain and stiffness in the joint. The treatments include physical therapy, radiofrequency ablation, non-steroidal anti-inflammatory drugs, anesthetic injection, and spine surgery. These treatments work differently and the doctor would decide which is best for the patient.

Some of these treatments may have side effects such as allergic reaction from the patient, bleeding, infection, paralysis, and even worsening of the pain. These side effects aren't common and the risks are higher in the 'anesthetic injection' treatment.

Osteoarthritis of the Spine

Osteoarthritis of the spine happens when there is a breakdown in the cartilage of the facet joint and the ligaments in the lower back and the neck. As a person grows older, the invertebrate disc can become dehydrated causing the disc to become narrow and adding more pressure to the facet joint.

The treatment centers on relieving the pain and increasing the patient's mobility. The condition itself is irreversible and there's no cure for it. Over-the-counter drugs may be used to relieve the pain. If they don't work, the doctor might prescribe antidepressants or may apply corticosteroid injection into the joint. Physical therapy, gentle exercises, and heat or cold therapy are other options.

The most common treatment is the use of over-the-counter drugs and they may come with side effects such as bleeding, upset stomach, or organ damage, especially if the patient doesn't use them as directed.

Subluxation

Subluxation refers to a misalignment in the position of the vertebrae in the spine. It leads to loss of functions due to different pressure points on the spinal column. It can be caused by a person's lifestyle or a traumatic event. A person that has a bad posture may have their spine shift out of alignment slowly, especially in areas of the soft tissue between the vertebrae.

The most common treatment is the chiropractic care which helps to restore the natural alignment of the spine. Other treatments include physical therapy, diet change, and regular exercising.

Side effects of chiropractic therapy include discomfort in the affected area and other pains, fatigue, nausea, dizziness, and other uncommonly reported individual reactions.

Spinal Stenosis

Spinal stenosis happens when the spinal column starts to narrow and compress the spinal cord. The process happens gradually and only causes problems when the narrowing is too much.

The treatment aims first at reducing the pain. Nonsteroidal anti-inflammatory drugs can be used. Injecting the spinal column with cortisone injections can also reduce the swelling. Physical therapy can also be used to stretch the body and strengthen the muscles. Surgery may be required if there's neurological loss or the pain is severe.

Some treatments require drugs with opioid quantities. This has to be carefully monitored because of several potentially serious side effects, including addiction. Steroid injections can also weaken the connective tissues and bones around the affected area. While surgery have less risks of complications, the surgeon's experience plays an important role.

Sciatica

Sciatica is a feeling of moderate to severe pain in the back, buttocks and legs (where the sciatic nerves run). It is caused by irritation of the nerve.

Common treatments of sciatica include using over-the-counter pain relief medication, stretching and regular exercises, cold and hot method, epidural steroid injection, surgery, and alternative treatments (like acupuncture, chiropractor and massage therapy).

Excessive use of aspirin and some over-the-counter pain relief medications can cause complications like ulcer and stomach bleeding. There are many side effects associated with epidural steroid injection, and this is why it's rarely offered.

Muscle Strain/Sprain

Muscle strain occurs when the muscles tear or are overstretched. It is caused by an improper or overuse of muscle or fatigue. Any muscle in the body can strain. But the most common muscle strains occur at the lower back, neck, hamstring, and shoulder. These strains can limit movement within the muscle group that they affect and they cause pain.

Muscle strain can be treated at home by resting, applying ice, compressing the muscle by applying bandage, and raising it above the level of the heart if possible. Patients can also use over-the-counter anti-inflammatory drugs. Also, they can engage in some exercises and stretch the muscle a little, while making sure they aren't resting it too much. They may also see a physical therapist. But if the muscle strain is severe, it's important to see a doctor. This is especially if the pain doesn't subside, the limbs can't move and the area is numb or has blood coming out. The use of NSAIDs is another treatment option.

The use of over-the-counter drugs may come with side effects like bleeding. There may also be serious medical conditions that may result from using NSAIDs if the patient have kidney or gastrointestinal disease.

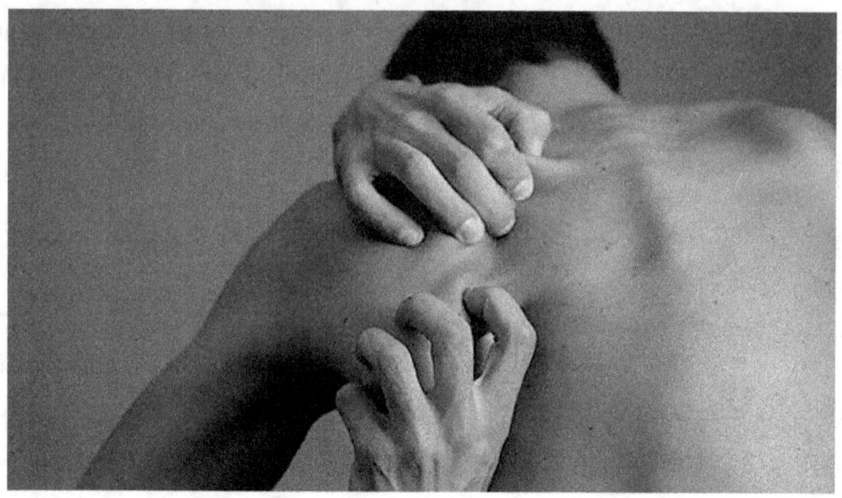

SHOULDER PAIN

The joint in the shoulder is the most mobile in the body including forward, backward, upward, and circular motion. There are different ways by which an individual can injure and start to feel pain in his shoulders. There are also certain diseases like cervical spine, heart, liver, and gallbladder diseases that can cause pain to the shoulder. The soft tissues around the shoulders might start to degenerate as one grows older. So, older people over the age of 60 are more prone to shoulder pain.

Rotator Cuff Tear

Rotator cuff muscles are the group of muscles and tendons that are responsible for stabilizing the shoulders. They also aid movement in the shoulder joint. It is also an area with a high tendency for injuries and tears. Rotator cuff tear is caused by an acute injury, or an overuse of the rotator cuff. The tendons connecting the muscles to the bones can tear partially or completely and this causes pain.

Treatments can vary from just resting the arm to undergoing surgery. Common treatments include using over-the-counter anti-inflammatory medication, resting the arm and wearing a sling over it, injecting it with cortisone to reduce inflammation, hot or cold therapy, exercises to restore the range of motion and strength. Surgery is quite unlikely for this pain.

Side effects of anti-inflammatory drugs include headache, upset stomach, vomiting, indigestion, constipation and ulcer. Cortisone injections can also have side effects like elevated blood sugar, weight gain, cataracts, and increased blood pressure.

GH Joint Arthritis

The acromiovascular joint and the glenohumeral joint are the two joints that make up the shoulder. The glenohumeral joint is where the humerus meets the scapula. This joint is quite prone to osteoarthritis, a degenerative joint disease in which the articular cartilage starts to wear out. This may lead to pain and swelling. This shoulder osteoarthritis is commoner in people over the age of 50. It can happen in younger people after a trauma or an injury such as dislocated shoulder or fracture.

Common treatments include using over-the-counter anti-inflammatory medication, resting the shoulder joint, hot or cold therapy, exercises to restore the range of motion and strength, physical therapy, and taking dietary supplement. Surgery is only necessary when these non-surgical treatments fail.

These treatment methods do not have any problems to them, except surgery, which has its own risks and complications may arise.

AC Joint Arthritis

The acromiovascular joint is where the scapula meets the collarbone. The wear and tear of cartilages around this area can lead to pain, swelling, and stiffness in the joint. This pain can limit the range of motion that the joint permits. This type of arthritis is commoner in older people.

Common treatments include using over-the-counter anti-inflammatory medication, resting the shoulder joint, hot or cold therapy, exercises to restore the range of motion and strength, physical therapy, injecting corticosteroid to reduce inflammation, and taking dietary supplement. Surgery is only necessary when these non-surgical treatments fail.

These treatment methods don't have any problems attached, except the injection of steroids which may have some side effects, which is why it is rarely used. Undergoing surgery also comes with its own risks and complications.

Labral Tear

The labrum is a soft cartilage around the socket joint in the shoulder bone.

The rotator cuff muscles help to keep the labrum in the socket, but injuries and repetitive motion can cause the labrum to tear and this can cause great pain.

Labral tear can be easily treated with some rest, physical therapy, and use of some over-the-counter medications. If it's a Bankart tear, the doctor would put the upper arm back in its place, after which the patient will go for physical therapy. Physical therapy is basically for strengthening the muscles around the shoulder, the rotator cuff especially. The person will also know the activities and positions to avoid or carry out. If the tear is severe, you might require surgery.

The non-surgical treatment for this pain doesn't have any problem. The problems might only arise from the risks and complications associated with surgery.

Biceps tendinopathy

Biceps tendinopathy is the inflammation of the tendon around the long head of the biceps muscle. It is more likely to occur in older people above 65years. It may also occur in athletes that are older in 35years as a result of sudden overuse.

The treatment of biceps tendinopathy is conservative but surgical if need be. NSAIDs are admitted for pain treatment followed by steroid injection if the pain persists. If the pains still remain, the patient can be injected with corticosteroid on the tendon sheath. If all of these conservative treatments prove unsuccessful, then surgical treatment comes in. But the first call is usually administration of medications, especially in medically complicated patients. Physical therapy is another common treatment of tendinopathy that should be pursued alongside the first two.

Not all biceps tendinopathy has an inflammatory nature, some are non-inflammatory. These non-inflammatory ones may not respond to cortisone injections or NSAIDs. In fact, they may even cause more complications in healing the tendinosis. The physiotherapist will have to recommend tendon strengthening exercises for such patient.

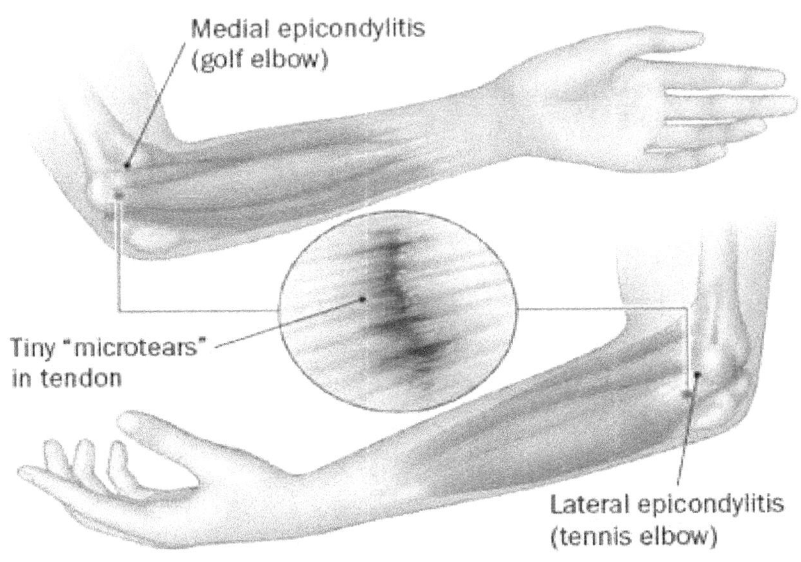

ELBOW PAIN

Elbow pain may occur as a result of several sporting injuries or simply from an overuse. Elbow pain may involve any of the following; arm muscles, tendons, elbow ligament, bursae, and bones in the arm. There are about 7 different elbow disorders and the sportsmen that are more prone to elbow pain are tennis players, baseball pitchers, golfers, and boxers.

Elbow Arthritis

Rheumatoid arthritis (RA) happens when the immune system is overactive. It affects both large and small joints in the body, developing especially in the elbow. When RA affects the elbow, it's often symmetrical, affecting both left and right arms. Elbow pain is often a sign of RA in its early stages.

The treatment is meant to reduce the stiffness, inflammation, and pain in the elbow. It doesn't cure the RA. The goal is usually to slow the disease's progression. Depending on the severity of the pain, treatments include both non-surgical and surgical options. Non-surgical options involve taking OTC pain medications, corticosteroids, disease-modifying anti-rheumatic drugs (DMARDs), and biologics. You could also apply cold or heat therapy, rest the joint, and attend physical therapy and occupational therapy. If the pain persists or the inflammation is uncontrolled, it may damage the elbow, and surgery would be required.

Side effects like upset stomach, diarrhea, nausea, hair loss, and organ problems may result from the use of DMARDs. There are also possible side effects to using OTC medication especially if it's not used properly.

Ulnar collateral ligament (UCL)

The inner part of the elbow has a ligament known as the ulnar collateral ligament. It is one of the two ligaments that help to prevent dislocation in the elbow, with the radial collateral ligament (RCL). The UCL is responsible for stabilizing the elbow while you throw, so it has to withstand a lot of stress. When the ligament tears, it's called a sprain and it causes pain. It can result from acute or chronic injury. There are 3 grades of sprain.

Conservative treatment of UCL sprain includes rest, physical therapy, anti-inflammatory drugs, and bracing. If the ligament tears completely or the pain persists after conservative treatment, surgery may be necessary.

There are no side effects to the conservative treatments except the use of anti-inflammatory drugs, in which case following the doctor's prescription is necessary. Surgery, on the other hand, can come with side effects like healing problems, nerve injury and infections.

Golfers Elbow

Golfers elbow is caused by wear and tear in the muscles, tendons, and bones in the elbow. It results from activities like repetitive gripping motions like weight lifting, rock climbing, racket sports, or throwing. This causes tenderness, pain and inflammation in the muscles in the inside part of the elbow.

Treatments include applying ice and resting the elbow, taking OTC anti-inflammatory drugs, bracing, practicing strengthening exercise, slowly returning to activities involving the arm. Doctors may recommend plasma-rich protein injections, or corticosteroid injection to relief the inflammation, or surgery if other conservative methods fail.

The treatment methods for golfers elbow are quite easy and aren't problematic. If patients take to doctor's prescription on the OTC drugs, they'll have no problems. But the corticosteroid injections may have some side effects. Surgery might not be necessary, but if it is, there's always a risk involved, with possible complications.

Tennis Elbow

When the tendons joining the forearm muscles and the outer part of the elbow together become inflamed, the condition is known as tennis elbow. Tennis players often develop this condition because of the repetitive use of the muscle, however, it's not exclusive to tennis players. It is mostly a problem of overuse of forearm muscles.

The treatment method is usually conservative and can be done at home. It includes rest, physical therapy, strapping the forearm, ice massage and muscle stimulating techniques, shock wave therapy, and steroid injection. In very rare cases, surgery may be required to relieve the pain if conservative treatment method does not in 6-12 months. There may be need to remove the damaged part of the tendon.

Using steroid injection may have side effects like shrinking of the fatty tissue at the site of the injection, loss of skin color at the injection site, pain on injection. It may also damage the tendon around the elbow, although it's rare. Shock wave therapy may also have side effects like short-term skin reddening, swelling at the treated area, and the treatment can also be painful.

Bursitis

Bursitis is an inflammation of the bursae surrounding the areas where muscle tissues, skin, and tendons meet the bones. The bursae lubricate these areas and help to reduce friction. When they become inflamed, it causes great pain and discomfort in that area and limit the movement of your joint.

Easy ways to relieve bursitis are resting, icing the affected joint, and taking pain medications. However, it's necessary to take antibiotics if the bursa becomes infected. Physical therapy is also important. Doctors may also inject the person wiith corticosteroids to relieve the pain and also reduce inflammation and swelling if it's not infected. Surgery becomes necessary if the bursae is damaged.

Side effects of taking bursa injection include swelling at the site of injection and bruising. Taking steroid medications may also have side effects such as flushed face, hiccups, slight fever, insomnia, headache, increased heart rate, water retention, increased appetite, and bloating.

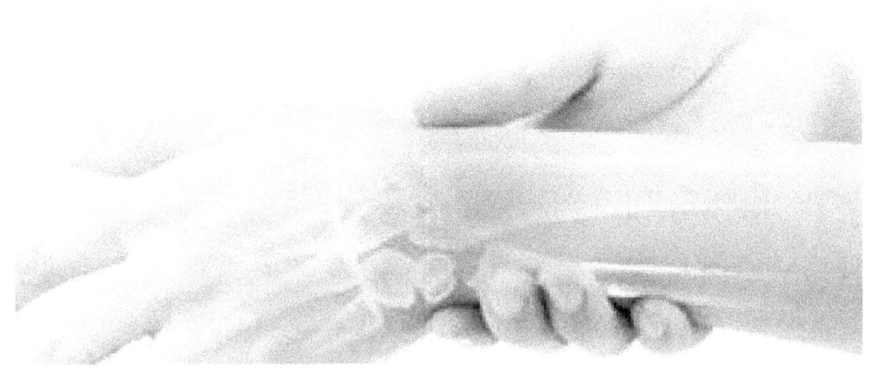

WRIST/HAND PAIN

The wrist is where the forearm bones and the hand bones meet. It isn't just a joint, it is several small joints meeting up. Wrist pain can result from sudden injury or impact. It can occur if a ligament becomes overstretched. It is caused by several other reasons. The wrist is important for basic movement and carrying out of day-to-day activities. Wrist pain can therefore affect the quality of a person's life.

Hand Osteoarthritis

Hand osteoarthritis may affect the wrist. It causes the cartilage between the joints to wear down, and the bones start to rub against each other. This rubbing causes pain, stiffness, and inflammation.

Common treatments may include taking OTC anti-inflammatory drugs, but if the OA is severe, the doctor may prescribe stronger drugs. Exercise is another common treatment that helps to maintain flexibility in the hands. Useful exercises include knuckle bends, fists, finger touches, and wall walking. Eating a more healthy diet with fruits and vegetables is also necessary. But if the OA doesn't respond to these treatments, surgery may become necessary.

Eating healthy and exercising has no side effects and if patients follow the doctor's prescription on the OTC drugs, they shouldn't experience any problems.

Hand Rheumatoid Arthritis

Rheumatoid arthritis is an autoimmune disease which makes the body attack its tissues. People suffering from RA are likely to suffer arthritis in their wrist making it hard for them to bend their wrist and perform daily activities after a while.

Rheumatoid arthritis doesn't have a cure, so treatment is centered on reducing pain, increasing mobility, and reducing joint damage. Initial treatment is to reduce pressure on the wrist and do little exercises. Doctors may recommend NSAIDs to control the inflammation. Other treatments include taking biologic drugs, pain killers, DMARDs, and corticosteroid injections.

Side effects like upset stomach, diarrhea, nausea, hair loss, and organ problems may result from the use of DMARDs. Corticosteroid injection may also come with some side effects.

CHAPTER: 13

NECK PAIN CONDITIONS

What are the common causes of neck pain?

Neck pain is a common medical condition, and various diseases and disorders may involve in this condition. Pain starts with dull aching, and sometimes it becomes worse with neck movement or during head-turning. Common symptoms of neck pain are associated with some other complaints including headache, muscle pain, tingling in arm, neck stiffness, fever, sore throat, arm weakness, numbness, sharp shooting pain, tenderness and motion difficulties, fullness, pulsation, difficulty in swallowing, swishing sound, dizziness, lymph node swelling and lightheadedness. The pain is also associated with some complicated symptoms, including shoulder pain, facial pain, and tingling. All of them are due to nerve pinching, and the severity of these symptoms may lead to back pain. Causative factors of neck pain are poorly understood and are typically multifactorial. These factors include neck strain, poor posture, depression and anxiety, occupational and sporting activities. Mechanical and degenerative factors are linked with chronic neck pain (Binder). Common causes of neck pain include poor posture, neck strain, neck injuries; including cervical radiculopathy (pinched nerve), herniated disc or whiplash, spinal stenosis, cervical spondylosis, osteoarthritis, or degenerative disc disease. Some infections, for example, a viral infection of the throat causes swelling of lymph node resulting in neck pain. Some rare infections also cause neck pain. These infections include Neck tuberculosis, spine bones infection in the neck (septic discitis and osteomyelitis), and meningitis (frequently escorted by neck stiffness). It can occur due to a direct effect on neck muscles. Such conditions include polymyalgia rheumatic and fibromyalgia, uncomfortable neck position at sleep (MedicineNet) (Bogdu)

How common is spinal degeneration/arthritis?

Spinal degeneration is common in many countries. About 19% of adults aged 45 to 64 and 57% of adults aged 65 and older suffer from arthritis in the United States (Alfred C. Gellhorn). 6 million people suffer from this disease in France. About 16% of the United States population suffers from arthritis (Reginster). About 21% of the US adults reported arthritis, 1.3 million have rheumatoid arthritis, and 2.4 milllion have spondylarthritides (Helmick). Between 1991 and 2031, the prevalence of arthritis diagnosed by any health professional in Canada increased from 10.7 to 15.7%, an increase of 46.7%, and the number of people with arthritis increased from 2.9 to 6.5 million, an increase of 124%. Comparable changes in prevalence and numbers of people with self-reported arthritis are 17.1% (4.7 million) to 23.6% (9.7 million). Most of the increase will be in the population aged 45+, and not until after 2020 will the corresponding increase in the 65+ age group be higher than that for the 45-64 age groups. Disability attributed to arthritis in the population aged 15+ is projected to increase from a prevalence of 2.3% (595,000) in 1991 to 3.3% (1.13 million) in 2031 (Badley EM).

When does it typically start (or why would it begin prematurely)

Typically it starts between 30-50years, but sometimes it begins in childhood because of calcium deficiency or any strain. Of people 18 to 44 years old, 7.3% report doctor-diagnosed arthritis, according to the CDC. Of people who are age 45–64, 30.3% report doctor-diagnosed arthritis. In the 65 or older age group, 49.7% report doctor-diagnosed arthritis. While the risk of developing most types of arthritis increases with age, keep in mind that it is not the only contributing factor. Among many causes of, the ageing process is most significant. With age comes the loss of fluid in the discs or cracks in the outer layer of the discs. Premature onset of this disease may occur with certain risky behaviours such as maintaining excessive body weight, engaging in heavy physical work, and even smoking (Health).

Treatment

First-line treatment for degenerative spine disease is conservative treatment. Therapy is useful until it will present acute neurological symptoms, including Cauda equine syndrome or myelopathy. Imaging and surgery will be considered if medication fails. Different approaches for surgery can be found, and it depends on the prevalent pattern of degeneration. Microdiscectomy is beneficial for symptomatic disc herniation (Kamper SJ). Surgical fusion is used for spinal stabilization if there is abnormal spinal motion or destabilization (McCrory DC). Interbody fusion implantation technique is used to support the anterior column and restore disc height (Hueng DY). However, spondylotic changes don't need any surgery (SergiyV.Kushchayev). Both surgery and medication can treat cervical spondylosis (arthritis of neck). However, the recommendation rate for surgery is relatively low for spondylolysis.

What is the standard of care to treat cervical spine conditions?

Cervical spine treatment follows a standard protocol which is initiated from initial stabilization and move towards the clinical examination. For treatment, steroid protocol is used, and surgery is the last option (O'Dowd). American health association makes a recommendation to treat cervical spine condition. There are four recommendations which are graded according to disease condition and required treatment protocol (Christopher M. Bono). These recommendations are

1. " 1- The diagnosis of cervical radiculopathy be considered in patients with arm pain, neck pain, scapular or periscapular pain, and paresthesias, numbness and sensory changes, weakness, or abnormal deep tendon reflexes in the arm. These are the most common clinical findings seen in patients with cervical radiculopathy."

2. 2- The diagnosis of cervical radiculopathy be considered in patients with atypical findings such as deltoid weakness, scapular winging, weakness of the intrinsic muscles of the hand, chest or deep breast pain, and headaches. Atypical symptoms and signs are often present in patients with cervical radiculopathy, and can improve with treatment."

3. 3- "Provocative tests, including the shoulder abduction and Spurling's tests, may be considered in evaluating patients with clinical signs and symptoms consistent with the diagnosis of cervical radiculopathy."

4. 4- Because dermatomal arm pain alone is insufficient in identifying the pathologic level in patients with cervical radiculopathy. Hence, further evaluation, including CT, CT myelography, or MRI, is suggested before surgical decompression."

What are the most commonly used therapies, drugs and

surgeries?

Treatment for degenerative spine diseases may include physical therapy, occupational therapy or combination of therapies, losing weight, medication and surgery. Few surgical options include Facet rhizotomy and IDET (Intradiscal electrothermal annuloplasty). ACDF, ADR and Posterior Cervical Laminoforaminotomy are also used surgical procedures. Drugs used to treat this condition include Acetaminophen, OTC and prescribed NSAIDs, antidepressant, neuropathic agents, muscle relaxants, steroid or opioid. Spinal injections include facet joint injection and Epidural steroid injection (Nordqvist) (Highsmith). Whereas, the medications for arthritis include; analgesics, NSAIDs, corticosteroids, **Traditional or targeted Disease-Modifying Antirheumatic Drugs and biologics (Foundation).**

What short and long-term complications are there using those treatments?

Short term use of aspirin and other NSAIDs are associated with colorectal neoplasia, opioid show drowsiness and constipation (World). While at long term use; risk of colorectal cancer is associated with dosage and duration (Andrew T. Chan). Long term use of NSAIDs and acetaminophen carry the risk factors for developing hematological malignancies (Roland B. Walter). Long term use of opioid causes opioid-induced hyperalgesia leads to increase pain sensitivity (Crofford). It also induces physical and psychological dependence in patients (World).

How likely will I get addicted to opioids if I use them to manage my neck pain?

Opioids use, according to doctor prescription, has a low risk of being an addict to those opioid, but few predisposing factors will influence on being an addict. Such factors include family or personal history of abuse substances or any psychiatric illness. The uncontrolled use of opioid leads to addiction, followed by tolerance and physical dependence. American health society defines terms. According to this; "Addiction has a genetic basis in addition to a psychological aspect to the behaviour. Addiction is associated with craving for the abused substance (such as an opioid), and continued, compulsive use of that substance despite harm to the person using the substance. In addition to having a genetic predisposition, there may be an environmental influence affecting both the development and manifestation of the addictive behaviour" (Medicine).

What are the surgical outcomes?

The success rates of ACDF surgery for neck pain caused by degenerative spines are 73-83% (Jewell).

How long can I expect my surgery to last?

Mostly surgery is done in 1-2 hours, but sometimes it can last for $2^{1/2}$ – 3hours. There is no standard protocol to determine how long a surgery lasts and time depends on diseases condition that how badly vertebrae or disc are affected (Healthcare).

What type of surgery is conducted most often for neck pain? How common is the need for revision surgery?

There are three surgical procedures to operate neck pain. These include Anterior Cervical Diskectomy and Fusion (ACDF), Artificial Disk Replacement (ADR) and Posterior Cervical Laminoforaminotomy. ACDF is most often used surgery for neck pain (Staurt J. Fischer). Patients after ACDF have a low chance of redevelopment, and there is a lesser need for revision surgery (Mohamad Bydon).

What conditions are 'high risk' if I have surgery? (Diabetes and COPD etc.)

Some patients are at high risk during operation and need special care. These may include older age patients (>70years old age), having any physiological reserve, severe cardio respiratory disorder like stroke, COPD or acute MI, last stage aortic disorder, previously done with surgery for carcinoma, acute massive blood loss, hemodynamic instability, septicaemia, septic focus or blood culture, acute renal or respiratory failure or diabetes (Jackson).

How successful is the utilization of post-surgical physical therapy in outcomes?

The results from literature reviews and prospective studies revealed that physiotherapy is considered necessary and post-operative physical therapy gives superior outcomes than others. Specific physical activities for after ACDF include endurance exercise, isometric strengthening and stretching. These are most appropriate for rehabilitation after ACDF (Leger).

How many disability claims in the United States are related to neck pain? How much money is spent on disability claims annually?

Social security disability insurance (SSDI) and supplemental security income (SSI) are the major disability claim in the United States related to neck pain. They come under the control of Social security administration

(SSA) (Help). Neck pain and lower back pain are the third-highest causes on which people spend. There is an estimation that people are paying $87.6billion (UI, $67.5billion-$94.1billion) annually till 2013 and nowadays, the estimated cost is $57.2billion (UI, $47.4billion-$64.4billion) due to lifestyle modification (Joseph L. Dieleman).

What should co-management with other doctors be done?

There are various examples of collaborating care given by different doctors, and it depends on the patient's clinical status. One doctor is chiropractor (the one who provide attention to spines), and other health professionals work together. Mostly a chiropractor and an osteopath doctor provide collaborative care depends on patient goal setting and supports by structured communication like telephonic consultation and record sharing. This collaborative care provided by co-management with other doctors facilitates active patient's involvement leads to decrease in radicular symptoms and improvement in living life (Michael B. Seidman).

What are the long term and short term complications after surgery?

There are various completions associated with spinal surgery. Some of them last for a short term while others are long term and lasts for a long time and sometimes that complication needs father surgery. Some complications are thrombophlebitis, lungs problems, infection, hardware fracture, implant migration, spinal cord injury, persistent pain, sexual dysfunction, transitional syndrome and pseudoarthrosis. Persistent pain is the dominant long term complication (Center).

How does Regenerative medicine offer an option to people instead of traditional drugs or surgery?

Pharmacologically, regenerative medicine offers the best treatment option as compared to traditional drugs or surgery because of some unique features. Some of them are

1. One can sufficiently recapitulate the complexity of the internal milieu to permit new functional tissue and organ formation in vitro for subsequent implantation in vivo.

2. Multiple bioactive compounds can be loaded into a sophisticated drug delivery system(s) that is locally placed to orchestrate a complete functional regenerative response.

3. Drugs can be targeted to specific nuclei in the brain (e.g., the center affected in Parkinson's disease) or any desired region(s) of organs/tissues to exert local therapeutic or healing effects (George J. Christ).

CHAPTER: 14

LOWER BACK PAIN CONDITIONS

What causes lower back pain?

Mostly back pain in the lower region (lumbar region) is due to any mechanical reason, and in most of the cases, it is associated with spondylosis (spinal degeneration). Some mechanical causes include strains and sprains, herniated disc or ruptured discs, intervertebral disc degeneration, sciatica, radiculopathy, traumatic injury, spondylolisthesis, skeletal irregularities or spinal stenosis. This pain rarely relates to serious underlying cause including infection, tumor, abdominal aortic aneurysms, equine cauda syndrome, kidney stones, and inflammatory disease of joints like arthritis, fibromyalgia, osteoporosis, and endometriosis (NINDS).

What types of conditions can occur (oa, ddd, herniation etc)

Low back pain can lead to various secondary complications as in the worst case. The patient may become bedridden, leading to blood clotting in legs and decrease muscle tone. Ultimately some other diseases occur as osteoarthritis or herniation. A herniation is rupturing of an intervertebral disc in which disc bulge out. This condition sometimes causes radiculopathy. (<u>NINDS</u>). The psychological complications associated with low back pain include depression and insomnia (<u>State</u>).

What is low back pain?

Almost every person experience this pain at any stage of life. The pain originates from the lumbar region (below the ribcage). Sometimes this pain becomes worse. This is a leading cause of missed work. The pain starts as dull muscle aches and changes into shooting or stabbing sensations. The movement will be painful or even in a straight standing position as the pain radiating down to legs and become worse when a person is lifting something, standing or bending or even in walking. Sometimes this pain improves with reclining. Acute pain comes suddenly mostly after heavy lifting or any injury from sports. If pain lasts for more than three months, it is considered as chronic pain (WebMD "Slideshow: A Visual Guide to Low Back Pain"; M. Clinic). Other symptoms that indicate serious health issue are: persistent fever, pain in abdomen with throbbing sensation, unexplained weight loss, intense pain at night, tingling or numbness in one or both legs and loss of urinary and bladder control (Lights and Leonard).

How common is it?

It is anticipated that lower back pain is one of the major injuries and diseases which accounts for the highest number of disability-adjusted life-years worldwide (<u>Vos et al.</u>). It is difficult to measure its incidence rate, particularly for its first episode as it is already high at adulthood and symptoms reappear over time. General Low back pain prevalence is 60-70 % in the industrially developed country from which 15-45% individuals are adults. And this rate is more economical in children and adolescents, but nowadays, this rate is also increasing (<u>Taimela et al.</u>; <u>Balague, Troussier</u>

and Salminen). Prevalence increases with age, and it is at a peak between 35-55years age (Andersson). According to Cleveland Clinic, about 80-90% of the United States population experience back pain at any stage of their life (State).

How is it treated?

First-line treatment for degenerative spine disease is conservative treatment. Therapy is useful until it will present acute neurological symptoms, including Cauda equine syndrome or myelopathy. Imaging and surgery will be considered if medication fails. Different approaches for surgery can be found, and it depends on the prevalent pattern of degeneration. Microdiscectomy is beneficial for symptomatic disc herniation (Kamper et al.). Surgical fusion is used for spinal stabilization if there is abnormal spinal motion or destabilization (McCrory et al.). Interbody fusion implantation technique is used to support the anterior column and restore disc height. However, spondylotic changes don't need any surgery. Both surgery and medication can treat spinal spondylosis. However, the recommendation rate for surgery is relatively low for spondylolysis (NINDS).

What does spinal degeneration mean?

Spinal degeneration is the conditions in which different degenerative changes occur in the spine that cause loss in normal spinal structure and functions. This condition is not typically associated with a specific injury, but age is also a factor of spinal degeneration. Repeated sprains, strains, and excessive use of the back cause a gradual degeneration of spinal discs. Almost everyone experiences some spinal disc degeneration after 40 years of age (C. Clinic).

How common is spinal degeneration and when does it typically start (or why would it start prematurely)

About 19% of adults age 45–64 years, and 57% of adults age 65 years suffer from spinal degeneration in the United States (Gellhorn, Katz and Suri). About 1.3milion and 1.75milion people suffer from such condition in England and Wales respectively. 6milion people suffer from this disease in France. About 16% of the United States population suffers from various types of spinal degeneration (Reginster). About 21% of the US adults reported arthritis, 1.3milion has rheumatoid arthritis, and 2.4 million have spondylarthritides (Hootman and Helmick). Between 1991 and 2031, the prevalence of arthritis diagnosed by any health professional in Canada will increase from 10.7 to 15.7%, an increase of 46.7%, and the number of people with arthritis will increase from 2.9 to 6.5 million, an increase of 124%. Comparable changes in prevalence and numbers of people with self-reported arthritis are 17.1% (4.7 million) to 23.6% (9.7 million). Most of the increase will be in the population aged 45+, and not until after 2020 will the corresponding increase in the 65+ age group be higher than that for the 45-64 age groups. Disability attributed to arthritis in the population aged 15+ is projected to increase from a prevalence of 2.3% (595,000) in 1991 to 3.3% (1.13 million) in 2031 (Badley and Wang). Commonly, low back pain starts at the age of 30-45 and become more common with age increase (NINDS). If it occurs at a young age, it is classified as non-specific low back pain and associated with headache or high physical activity. The other possible reason is the gap between their physical activity capability and social needs of being physically active (Taguchi).

What types of treatments are available: surgery, pt, chiro, accupuncture, massage, stretches, pain management, opiods, nerve ablations/ blocks, arthritis meds, anti-inflammatory, steroids?

What are their outcomes?

Different treatment options are available for low back pain, which include medication, surgery, and physical therapy. Some of them are discussed here. Conventional treatment includes increasing physical activity, use of hot and cold bags, strengthening exercises. While medications include anti-inflammatory agents, steroids and opioids but their long term use also causes some complication. The use of opioid may cause addiction or dependence if it is used without strict monitoring of a physician. Other treatment options include spinal manipulation, which comes under the category of chiropractic care where doctors use his hands to adjust, massage, mobilize, and stimulate degenerative spine. This technique gives small to moderate relief for short term and is not affected if the patient has arthritis, spinal cord compression, or osteoporosis. Traction is a method which involves the use of pulleys and weights to provide constant pull to skeletal muscle, but when pressure is released, pain tends to return quickly and give temporary relief. Acupuncture is done by thin needles insertion throughout the body into precise points and is moderately helpful for chronic pain. Biofeedback therapy involves electrodes attached to the skin, and an electromyography machine is used to allow people to self-regulate their skin temperature, muscle tension, breathing, and heart rate. They regulate their pain response with relaxation techniques. This therapy is mostly used in combination and doesn't have side effects. There is no substantial evidence about the efficiency of this therapy. A nerve block therapy is used for chronic pain in which it blocks nerve conduction from specific body areas. Its success depends on the practitioner's ability to situate and inject the correct nerve accurately. Constant use of this practice leads to enhance functional impairment. Transcutaneous electrical nerve stimulation (TENS) involves taking a battery-powered device having electrodes and placed on the skin over the painful part. It generates electrical impulses intended to block incoming pain signals from peripheral nerves. It is useful for low back pain (NINDS).

What is the standard of care to treat cervical spine conditions?

Cervical spine treatment follows a standard protocol which is initiated from initial stabilization and move towards the clinical examination. For treatment, steroid protocol is used, and surgery is the last option (O'Dowd). American health association makes a recommendation to treat cervical spine condition. There are four recommendations which are graded according to disease condition and required treatment protocol (Bono et al.). These recommendations are

1- "The diagnosis of cervical radiculopathy is considered in patients with arm pain, neck pain, scapular or periscapular pain, and paresthesias, numbness and sensory changes, weakness, or abnormal deep tendon reflexes in the arm. These are the most common clinical findings seen in patients with cervical radiculopathy."

2- "The diagnosis of cervical radiculopathy is considered in patients with atypical findings such as deltoid weakness, scapular winging, weakness of the intrinsic muscles of the hand, chest or deep breast pain, and headaches. Atypical symptoms and signs are often present in patients with cervical radiculopathy, and can improve with treatment."

3- "Provocative tests, including the shoulder abduction and Spurling's tests, may be considered in evaluating patients with clinical signs and symptoms consistent with the diagnosis of cervical radiculopathy."

4- "Dermatomal arm pain alone is insufficient in identifying the pathologic level in patients with cervical radiculopathy. Hence, further evaluation, including CT, CT myelography, or MRI, is suggested before surgical decompression."

What drugs and surgeries are most commonly used?

Treatment for degenerative spine diseases may include physical therapy, occupational therapy, or a combination of therapies, losing weight, medication, and surgery. Few surgical options include artificial disc replacement, spinal fusion, radiofrequency denervation, plasma disc decompression (PDD) or nucleoplasty, Intradiscal electrothermal therapy (IDET), Foraminotomy, Discectomy or microdiscectomy, Spinal laminectomy or spinal decompression, Vertebroplasty and kyphoplasty. Drugs used to treat this condition include Acetaminophen, OTC (ibuprofen, ketoprofen, and naproxen sodium) and prescribed NSAIDs, antidepressant tricyclics and serotonin and norepinephrine reuptake inhibitors, neuropathic agents, muscle relaxants, steroid or opioid (codeine, oxycodone, hydrocodone, and morphine) and counter irritants. Nerve blocking and epidural steroidal injection are also used for low back pain (NINDS).

What types of conditions do people have that make them a bad candidate for surgery? (i.e: Diabetes, COPD, old age)

Some patients are at high risk during operation and need special care. These may include older age patients (>70years old age), having any physiological reserve, severe cardiorespiratory disorder like stroke, COPD or acute MI, last stage aortic disorder, previously done with surgery for carcinoma, acute massive blood loss, hemodynamic instability, septicaemia, septic focus or blood culture, acute renal or respiratory failure or diabetes (Boyd and Jackson).

What short and long-term complications are there using

those treatments?

There are various completions associated with spinal surgery. Some of them last for a short term while others are long term and lasts for a long time, and sometimes that complication needs father surgery. Some complications are thrombophlebitis, infection, lungs problems, implant migration, hardware fracture, persistent pain, spinal cord injury, pseudoarthrosis, transitional syndrome, and sexual dysfunction. Persistent pain is the dominant long term complication. NSAIDs has more potential to cause complication on long term use. These complications include heartburn, stomach irritation, diarrhea, ulcer, fluid retention, or in rare cases; these may cause cardiovascular diseases or kidney dysfunction (Nasser et al.; NINDS).

How long is the down time after surgery before one can be back to work?

Mostly surgery is done in 1-2 hours, but sometimes it can last for 21/2 – 3hours. There is no standard protocol to determine how long a surgery lasts and time depends on diseases condition that how badly vertebrae or disc are affected (Cherry). The recovery depends on overall health and degree of spinal degeneration. Spinal fusion takes about 6months for recovery while the procedure of discectomy takes 12weeks after surgery for making a person able to go back to his work (WebMD "Tips to Help You Recover from Back Surgery").

How often are opioids prescribed for back pain?

For treating low back pain, the opioid prescription is increasing, and now it is the most commonly prescribed drug. Opioid prescribing rate is two-three times higher in Canada and the United States than in Europe (Deyo, Von Korff and Duhrkoop).

How likely will I get addicted to opioids if I use them to manage my pain?

Opioids use, according to doctor prescription, has a low risk of being an addict to those opioid, but few predisposing factors will influence on being an addict. Such factors include family or personal history of abuse substances or any psychiatric illness. The uncontrolled use of opioid leads to addiction, followed by tolerance and physical dependence. American health society defines terms. According to this; "Addiction has a genetic basis in addition to a psychological aspect to the behavior. Addiction is associated with craving for the abused substance (such as an opioid), and continued, compulsive use of that substance despite harm to the person using the substance. In addition to having a genetic predisposition, there may be an environmental influence affecting both the development and manifestation of the addictive behavior" (ASRA).

What are the surgical outcomes success rates failure rates?

The success rate of the degenerative spine for low back pain is 80-90% for spinal fusion, and it depends on the patient's condition (Ullrich).

How long can I expect my surgery to last?

Mostly surgery is done in 1-2 hours, but sometimes it can last for 21/2 – 3hours. There is no standard protocol to determine how long a surgery lasts and time depends on diseases condition that how badly vertebrae or disc are affected (Cherry).

What type of surgery is conducted most often for back pain?

There are many types of surgeries for back pain including artificial disc replacement, spinal fusion, radiofrequency denervation, plasma disc decompression (PDD) or nucleoplasty, Intradiscal electrothermal therapy (IDET), Foraminotomy, Discectomy or microdiscectomy, Spinal laminectomy or spinal decompression, Vertebroplasty and kyphoplasty (NINDS). Among them, spinal fusion and spinal laminectomy (spinal decompression) are the most commonly used surgeries for low back pain (WebMD "Back Surgery: Pros and Cons").

Importance of pre and/or post-surgical rehabilitation?

Surgical rehabilitation is associated with counseling and physical therapy. Pre-Surgical Physical Therapy is needed to Mentally prepare the patient, Restore motion range, decrease pain and inflammation, enhance muscle control, normalize patterns of movement, Improve overall fitness while Post-Surgical Physical Therapy is vital to reduce swelling, regain motion range and lost strength, increased endurance and return to daily activities (Drayer).

How many disability claims in the United States are related to back pain?

With a rise in world population age, low back pain increases as intervertebral disc deterioration occur in older age. The pain is leading cause of limited activity and absence from work throughout the whole world and imposes a high economic burden on country's economy as its effects on all including, the person himself, his family, industry, and government as well (Taimela et al.; Andersson). In the United States, about 149milion workdays are lost because of low back pain (Guo et al.) with an estimated annual loss of 100-200billion US$ (Katz; Rubin). Social security disability insurance (SSDI) and supplemental security income (SSI) are the major disability claim in the United States related to back pain. They come under the control of Social security administration (SSA) (Help). Lower back pain and neck pain are the third-highest causes on which people spend. There is an estimation that people are paying $87.6billion (UI, $67.5billion-$94.1billion) annually till 2013 and nowadays, the estimated cost is $57.2billion (UI, $47.4billion-$64.4billion) due to lifestyle modification (Dieleman et al.).

What are the long term and short term complications after surgery, success rates of spinal fusion surgery, and % of revision surgeries?

There are various completions associated with spinal surgery. Some of them last for a short term while others are long term and lasts for a long time, and sometimes that complication needs father surgery. Some complications are thrombophlebitis, infection, lungs problems, implant migration, hardware fracture, persistent pain, spinal cord injury, pseudoarthrosis, transitional syndrome, and sexual dysfunction. Persistent pain is the dominant long term complication (Nasser et al.). The success rate of the degenerative spine for low back pain is 80-90% for spinal fusion, and it depends on the patient's condition (Ullrich). In lumbar spinal surgery, failure risk is 37% without spinal fusion and 30% with spinal fusion. Careful selection of surgical technique decreases the chance of the need for revision surgery. Otherwise, it is needed after one year (Eichholz and Ryken).

CHAPTER: 15

UPPER LIMB CONDITIONS

Introduction

In the upper limb, work-related musculoskeletal problems have an expansive scope of medical issues related to repetitive and strenuous work. These medical issues run from distress, minor throbbing and painfulness, to progressively genuine diseases which can prompt serious disabilities. Consistently a great many European laborers are influenced by musculoskeletal diseases of the upper limb. It is mostly connected with manual handling and with work reiteration and unbalanced work stances and postures. The work-related disorders and those issues which are caused by repetitive movement of the Upper Limb can influence any area of the neck, shoulders, arms, lower arms, wrists, and hand. Some of them are tendonitis, carpal tunnel disorder, Osteoarthritis, Adhesive Capsulitis (Frozen Shoulder) which have well-characterized signs and manifestations, while others are less well-characterized, including just pain, inconvenience, tingling, numbness, and discomfort. The upper limb disorders associated with neck problems are defined by Upton's and McComas hypothesis of "double-crush syndromes". The hypothesis was formulated in 1973; according to it, the patients having carpal tunnel syndrome not only have compressive lesions at the wrist but there is also some definite damage at the region of cervical nerve roots. (Upton)

What are common conditions that affect upper extremity (shoulder, elbow, wrist, hand)?

The most common conditions that affect the upper extremity and are encountered in the practice of medical specialties such as neurology, orthopedic surgery, rheumatology, and rehabilitation are as under:

Table 1: Classification of most common conditions that affect upper limb:

Shoulder	Adhesive Capsulitis (Frozen Shoulder)	
	Rotator Cuff disorders	
	Bicipital Tendinitis	
	Glenohumeral Arthritis	
Elbow	Olecranon Bursitis	
	Epicondylitis	
	Tenosynovitis- Extensor pollicis longus flexors	

Wrist/ Hand	Carpal Tunnel Syndrome	
	Arthritis	

<u>Shoulder</u>

- Adhesive Capsulitis

The cause of adhesive capsulitis is unclear; however, it is a situation that causes chronic pain of the shoulder. In this condition, the capsule of the shoulder (connective tissue around the glenohumeral joint of the shoulder) undergoes inflammation and becomes hard/stiff. The motion of the shoulder becomes highly restricted in this condition causing discomfort to the patient.

- Rotator Cuff Disorder

The rotator cuff disorder is a collection of disorders in which either the tendon or the bursa of the shoulder become inflamed, and the tissues of the shoulder are damaged, causing discomfort and pain to the patient.

- Bicipital tendinitis

In the bicipital tendinitis, the long head of the biceps undergoes inflammation. This disorder of the shoulder is prevalent because of the location and function of the bicep tendon.

- Glenohumeral Arthritis

In this condition, the narrowing of the glenohumeral joint takes place because of degeneration of the articular cartilage of the shoulder. It is also known as degenerative shoulder osteoarthritis, and it's a very painful condition.

Elbow

- Olecranon Bursitis

It is the inflammation of the bursa of the elbow. It is the most common type of bursitis and causes severe pain at the tip of the elbow.

- Epicondylitis

It is the inflammation of the tendons present around the elbow. There are two types of the epicondylitis, i.e., lateral epicondylitis, also known as tennis elbow and medial epicondylitis, also known as golfer's elbow. The epicondylitis occurs by repetitive movement of the elbow and forearm.

Wrist/ Hand

- Tenosynovitis

This disorder is called de Quervain's tenosynovitis. It occurs at the level of the radial styloid process. In this condition, tendons of abductor pollicis longus and extensor pollicis brevis get inflamed and swelled.

- Carpal Tunnel Syndrome

The carpal tunnel syndrome is a condition in which the median nerve impinges as it passes through the wrist. It causes severe pain and numbness in hand and arm.

What are the typical treatments of conditions discussed above?

The conditions discussed above are mainly related to soft tissues, i.e., inflammation of tendons, bursa, connective tissue, articular cartilage, etc.

The conservative management of soft tissue disorders is mostly preferred over invasive procedures, for example, surgery. However, if a grade III tear of soft tissue occurs, then surgery is the only option for treatment.

- So, first of all, modification of the workplace is needed to minimize the physical activity causing these issues.

- Some physical therapies can be used which includes soft tissue mobilization, exercise, stretching, ultrasound, splinting, TENS, local heat, Short wave diathermy, myofascial release technique, etc.

- Local injections of corticosteroids can also be given.

- Non-steroidal anti-inflammatory drugs (NSAIDs) can be used to treat symptoms and relieve pain.

- Surgery, in case of severe soft tissue injury.

What are the outcomes of the treatments?

The outcomes of the treatments vary patient to patient depending upon their ages and severity of the disorder. However, conservative treatment has shown significant improvements lessening the need to undergo invasive procedures. According to Giele et al., (H.) in the case of carpal tunnel syndrome, taking steroids reduced the symptoms. In another study (Gerritsen AA) proved that local injection significantly improved the symptoms of carpal tunnel syndrome at one month.

In the case of epicondylitis, conservative management has been beneficial in reducing the symptoms. According to a study, (Hay EM), to treat lateral epicondylitis, local steroid injections have shown noticeable results; however, the use of topical NSAIDs gave relief to some patients in the short-term as identified by (Green S). Physiotherapy also relieves the symptoms greatly over one year in case of epicondylitis. (Smidt N).

In a study conducted by Bartolozzi (Bartolozzi A), patients of rotator cuff syndrome and bicipital tendonitis were given combined treatments, i.e., local steroid, physical therapy, and NSAIDs. Around 46% of patients experienced significant improvements at six months of conservative management. Shoulder adhesive capsulitis has also been treated by the help of conservative management. According to a study, (Gam AN), patients who had symptoms of the frozen shoulder for more than six weeks, the pain worsened at night, and the range of motion was restricted; the injection of glucocorticoid brought significant improvement in functional movement.

How effective is treating carpal tunnel syndrome with surgery?

The aim of the surgery in the case of carpal tunnel syndrome is to reduce pressure on the median nerve. The surgery in CTS is typically possibly considered if there is a consistent return of the symptoms and if issues related to the excruciating pain increase. If the symptoms don't improve in spite of using conservative management, for example, corticosteroid injections, physiotherapy, splints, etc. then in those cases surgery can give preferable help over recurrent injections or support medicines. Carpal Tunnel syndrome does not happen suddenly. It mostly takes place after some damage, bleeding, or infection in the area of the wrist. In such cases, surgery is the only option.

Most people get relief after surgery. The symptoms improve significantly if the patient does not feel any abnormal sensations in the wrist, following surgery. The recovery after surgery depends upon the severity of impingement of the median nerve. It can take a little while or months for increasingly extreme indications to leave totally. After the surgery, the pain improves; however, the unusual sensations might take long to be treated thoroughly.

In some cases, the surgery for CTS does not help. The symptoms may not leave, or may return after that. It is hard to foresee how successful surgery will be. This may rely upon things like to what extent you have had manifestations and how extreme they are, or whether you have other health issues. The odds of achievement are higher if the condition is in a prior stage. According to a study (Huisstede BM), the symptoms have been improved in around 75 to 90% of individuals who were in an earlier stage. They even reported being symptom-free after some years. However, the CTS can be treated without surgery as well.

How many cases of carpal tunnel syndrome also have cervical spine involvement?

Dr. Adrian Upton, in his research tried to explain why the patients having Carpal tunnel syndrome also experience other issues such as pain in their shoulder, upper back, upper arm, forearm, and elbow. If the patients experience pain in different locations other than the wrist then only 10% of them would have a problem in their wrist. The problem is present in the region of the cervical spine where there might be irritation or impingement of the nerve root. The word "syndrome" has been used for it because neck problems also contribute to it.

The involvement of the cervical spine issue along with carpal tunnel has been named "Double crush syndrome". The hypothesis of double crush syndrome was constructed in 1973. According to the hypothesis, if the axons have been compressed on one end, they will be damaged at the other end. (Upton)In his study, utilized 115 patients, out of which 81 cases were found to have neural lesions in the cervical spine. Further studies were conducted in 1981 by Massey's, and he found 19 instances of CTS who also had cervical radiculopathy.

(Note – Dr. Adrian R.M Upton along with his co-worker AlanJ Mccomas worked on "double-crush syndrome" in 1973. Upton belongs to

Department of Medicine (Neurology). He worked at McMaster University Medical Centre, Hamilton, Ontario, Canada. Upton has worked on a few more projects which includes, deep brain stimulation as a treatment for refractory epilepsy, Aneurysmal subarachnoid hemorrhage prognostic decision-making algorithms, Alterations in the brain-body interface in aneurysmal subarachnoid hemorrhage, etc.)

How often does a shoulder joint replacement occur in the USA?

As per the Agency for Healthcare Research and Quality, currently, around 53,000 individuals in the U.S. have total shoulder arthroplasty every year. It makes it more than 900,000 Americans per year who have knee and hip arthroplasties. (Kiet)

What factors may be present that prevent a patient from being unable to have a Joint Replacement? (Age, diabetes, bone density, COPD, cardiovascular diseases .etc.)

Patients with diabetes might be unable to have a joint replacement as it has adverse effects on joint health. If a diabetic patient undergoes a surgical procedure, then proper the management of blood glucose levels is required first. Ignorance regarding the management of blood glucose levels can put a diabetic patient at high risk of postoperative complications. The diabetic patients are at high risk of having peri-prosthetic infection soon after joint replacement surgery. As a result of the research conducted by National Institutes of Health Clinical Translational Science Award 1 KL2 RR024151-01 (Mayo Clinic Center for Clinical and Translational Research) on total shoulder arthroplasty (TSA), due to diabetes around 9.4% of the patients developed a post-surgical infection.

In the elderly, osteoarthritis is widespread, affecting their quality of life and making them more in need of having arthroplasty. However, the osteoarthritis and osteoporosis can co-exist, leading to complications during arthroplasty. The osteoporosis or reduced bone density can have a problem with joint replacement surgeries. The problems include implant migration, intraoperative fracture of the bone, postoperative peri-prosthetic fracture. All of these problems can further affect the quality of life of the patients.

COPD is a common disease, and its occurrence increment with age. The degenerative changes in upper extremities additionally increment with increasing age. Along these lines, COPD patients are more in need of having upper extremities' joint replacement surgery. After the failure of conservative management, joint replacement stays as the mainstay of treatment. However, during arthroplasty, the COPD patients can have high serum C-reactive protein and leukocytes preoperatively and need of the red blood cells transfusions. The COPD patients will more now and again be admitted to the emergency unit; they might have high chances of wound infections, and the longer hospitalization time. They might even have pneumonia. So, COPD patients can have various problems if they undergo joint replacement surgery of the upper limb.

What is the risk of infection, amputation, death from total shoulder and elbow replacement surgery?

The total shoulder arthroplasty (TSA) has become a common surgery after the success of total hip and knee arthroplasty. The patients having severe or end-stage shoulder joint arthritis ultimately need total shoulder arthroplasty (TSA). The patients, after undergoing the TSA experience improvement in their pain, movement, and function of the shoulder, and quality of life. The chance of development of infection after TSA is very uncommon. According to a study, the incidence of infection has been reported ranging between .4%5 and 2.9%. As per a 20-year follow up, the rate of infection was low in patients of TSA. The causative agents of deep periprosthetic infections in TSA are mainly *Staphylococcus* and

Propionibacterium. According to the research conducted at Mayo Clinic Center for Clinical and Translational Research on total shoulder arthroplasty, after TSA male gender and younger aged patients are at higher risk of developing deep periprosthetic infections.

Total shoulder replacement and hemiarthroplasty have turned out to be acknowledged treatment choices for a different shoulder issue. During the previous 30 years, a more noteworthy comprehension of the biomechanics of shoulder function, related to better prosthetic structure, has diminished the complexities related with a shoulder replacement. Be that as it may, the infection has stayed one of the most crushing inconveniences requiring amendment medical procedure. The commonness of profound periprosthetic infection, including shoulder arthroplasty is accounted for somewhere in the range of 0% and 3.9% for unconstrained shoulder arthroplasties and 0% and 15.4% for obliged arthroplasties.

The mortality rate during or after the total shoulder arthroplasty (TSA) is extremely low. In between 2005 and 2011, the incidence of in-patient mortality for the patients undergoing the procedure of Total shoulder arthroplasty was less than 1 in 1000 surgeries. (White). There is a lack of information on the risk of amputation from total shoulder arthroplasty (TSA).

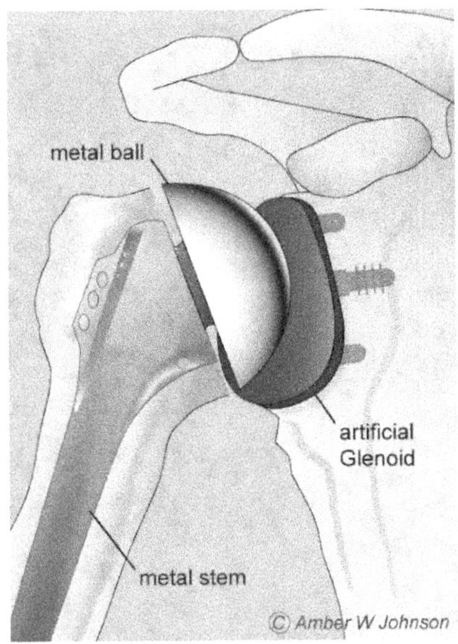

Figure 1: Total Shoulder Arthroplasty

https://www.google.com/url?sa=i&url=https%3A%2F%2Fwww.oamkg.com%2Fspecialties%2F
shoulder-
elbow.html&psig=AOvVaw3LP7HTil5EV2gJNAB9llDA&ust=1569074479117000&source=ima
ges&cd=vfe&ved=0CAIQjRxqFwoTCNCL6IXI3-QCFQAAAAAdAAAAABAE

In the case of total elbow arthroplasty (TEA), infection is one of the most serious complications. According to the studies, the rate of infection is as high as 11% in patients of TEA. And through more recent studies, the rate of infection in TEA patients has been reported to be between 2-5%. However, the rates on infection in TEA are higher as compared to hip and knee arthroplasties. The risk factors that contribute to the development of infection comprise diabetes mellitus, oral steroid use, and osteomyelitis. Infection may also develop in case the patient had a history of septic arthritis anywhere near the affected elbow.

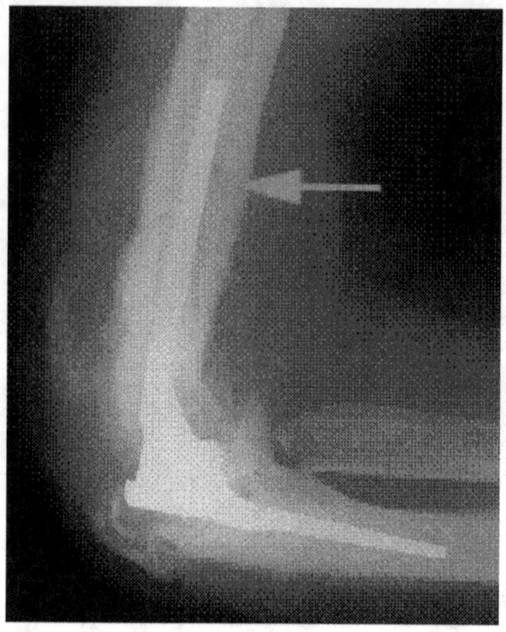

Figure2: Image of the infected elbow joint after Total Elbow Arthroplasty (TEA) (Red arrow shows large joint effusion)

The risk of death after total elbow arthroplasty is low. Mostly, the elder patients having certain comorbidities or the patients who had TEA after traumatic distal humeral fracture become victims of death.

What is the risk of clots or complications?

The total shoulder arthroplasty (TSA) and total elbow arthroplasty (TEA) are major surgeries in which the patients are put under general anesthesia. Therefore, there is a very low risk of heart attack, stroke, or even blood clots. If the blood clots are formed in the deep veins, it is called deep venous thrombosis (DVT). However, DVT most commonly occurs in lower limbs rather than upper extremities.

If the blood clot forms and left untreated, then it can dislodge from the wall of vessels leading to pulmonary embolism, which is a life-threatening condition. If the blood lot is treated timely, the patient can be prevented from pulmonary embolism through anti-clotting drugs such as heparin. In the case of shoulder and elbow arthroplasties, there is a low risk of formation of a blood clot. One thorough examination uncovered that among 42,261 shoulder-replacement surgeries, around 0.52% of patients (or around 220 individuals) encountered a blood clot post-medical procedure. (OjIKE) Luckily the complications rate after the medical procedure is little (under five percent).

What limitation exists post-surgery?

After the total shoulder arthroplasty (TSA) or total elbow arthroplasty (TEA), the patient must avoid the following things:

- The patient must not lift heavy objects with the affected arm without supporting it through the sound arm.

- In the early days, the patient is supposed to move their arm to a limited range (ROM becomes limited).

- The patient should avoid unnecessary above-head movements of the shoulder or elbow.

- Six weeks after the total elbow arthroplasty, the patient is advised not to pull anything towards them, for example, opening the door, or pulling their pants.

- The patient is not supposed to make sudden jerking movements with the affected arm.

- The patient is advised not to do the activities that have repeated movements such as weight lifting.

- After the TSA or TEA jamming or pounding activities, such as hammering, is prohibited.

- The patients cannot take part in sports like boxing.

What is the typical rehab and downtime required?

The patient is sent back home with a bandage and stitches which are removed as per the advice of the surgeon. If the patient has staples on the incision, then the surgeon will evacuate them in 10 to 21 days. In case of stitches, the surgeon will remove them in 10 to 14 days. The patient might feel tenderness, and pain and there might be some swelling in the region soon after the procedure. The primary care physician will give medication for the pain.

The rehabilitation program starts on the day of surgery. The physical therapist guides the patient regarding appropriate movement and exercise. The more the patient is focused on the recovery program, the sooner he will recover his quality of life and development. The downtime of the procedure is approximately 2 to 3 weeks which may vary depending upon the age of the patient. The rehabilitation program is then progressed towards strengthening exercises of the arm.

How often are steroids used to treat extremities?

The steroids are most commonly prescribed by the physicians to treat the rheumatologic diseases of the upper extremities. The most common steroid which is prescribed for this purpose is prednisone. It works rapidly and gives rapid relief to the patients as it reduces inflammation.

How successful are steroids?

Steroids have been proved to be very successful because of their ability to treat inflammation. Steroids act as cortisol which is a hormone produced naturally by our bodies. Despite its side effects, steroids are beneficial in dealing with critical situations in which most essential organs of the body such as kidney are in danger. The use of steroids in case of arthritis can give rapid relief to the patients.

What is the risk of using steroids over time?

The risk of using steroids over time is that it suppresses the hypothalamic-pituitary axis and can cause several different infections. The excessive use of steroids can lead to dermatologic changes, systemic problems such as Cushing's syndrome, cardiovascular problems which can create life-threatening conditions, ophthalmologic problems, and problems related to GIT, weakness of bone and muscle, neuropsychiatric issues leading to depression, suppression of immune system, metabolic and endocrine issues and many more.

What is the occurrence of repeat procedures?

In the USA, the occurrence of re-operation of total elbow arthroplasty is only 0.5% which can occur due to complications. (Van Riet)

What is the life expectancy after an older person has shoulder replacement Surgery?

Total shoulder arthroplasty is an exceptionally successful procedure, and the ten survival rate is up to 90 percent. Total shoulder arthroplasty can be performed in patients 80 years and more established with paces of perioperative complexities and mortalities similar to those of more youthful patients, in spite of the fact that these more elderly patients may require a more drawn out time of institutional consideration before come back to home and might be bound to need a blood transfusion.

Effectiveness of treating neuropathy in hands with medication? Risks and benefits? I.e.: (gabapentin

In the neuropathy in hands such as Carpal Tunnel Syndrome which is caused due to impingement of the median nerve, the use of gabapentin is a very effective treatment. The benefits of using gabapentin for carpal tunnel syndrome constitute the ability to pinch, grip and decrease in abnormal sensations in the wrist. If administered in low doses, gabapentin is useful in the treatment of Carpal tunnel syndrome without any side effects. Use of 300 mg/ day is more effective as compared to 100 mg/day. However, if administered in as high as 900-1800 mg/day, gabapentin becomes intolerable by some patients. (Duman). The side effects include abnormal eye movements, difficulty speaking, diarrhea, dry mouth, nausea.

CHAPTER: 16

LOWER LIMB CONDITIONS

What are the common conditions that affect these areas?

Hip pain is a general complaint which occurs due to a wide variety of problems. Pain on the outer side of the hip, outer buttock or upper thigh is generally caused by problems associated with muscles, ligaments, tendons, and other soft tissues that surround the hip joint. Ankle pain refers to any pain or discomfort in ankles. Pain and tenderness, associated with plantar fascia strains and usually felt on the bottom of the foot between the heel and the base of the toes, are referred to as foot pain. While knee pain is confined to pain at the knee joint usually due to injury. Some common causes of lower extremity pain are:

- Hip pain after unreasonable sitting or leaning over a PC for a considerable length of time at once.

- Foot and knee pain after standing, bowing, or being in an "inappropriate position".

- Knee and lower leg pain after constant stress, for example, transferring a substantial pack or handbag.

Temporary knee pain often leads to permanent knee pain. Many individuals experience temporary knee pain because of damage or mishap. Unending knee pain once in a while leave without treatment, and it does not stop. It's regularly the consequence of a few causes or conditions.

Physical conditions or illnesses can cause knee pain, which include:

- Osteoarthritis: pain, disturbance, and joint obliteration achieved by degeneration and disintegrating of the joint

- Tendinitis: pain in the front of the knee that is disturbed when climbing, taking stairs, or walking around an incline.

- Chondromalacia patella: damaged tendon under the kneecap.

- Gout: joint irritation recognized by uric acid.

- Dough strong development: an advancement of synovial (a fluid that oils up the joint) behind the knee.

- Rheumatoid joint pain: a determined hard framework critical issue that causes painful swelling and can at last reason joint deformation and bone deterioration.

- Withdrawal: partition of the kneecap as often as possible the outcome of damage.

- Meniscus tear: a burst at any rate in one of the tendons in the knee.

- Torn tendon: tear in one of the four ligaments in the knee — the most ordinarily hurt ligament is the anterior cruciate ligament (ACL).

- Bone tumors: osteosarcoma (second most unavoidable bone threat), most ordinarily occurs in the knee.

What are the run of the mill medicines?

Hip Injuries

Hip injuries can consolidate tissue, bone, and injuries. Pain in the hip can be escaped from the spine plate and nerve wounds. The pelvic bones, for the most part, genital pulls, and hernias can reduce hip joint injuries. Hip pain is commonly limited to the genital zone. The isolation of the backside can be related to acrylic joint injuries and distress apparently of the hip can be related to hip crack and surplus gluteus medius tears.

Pain from inside the hip joint, regularly genital pain can consolidate hip tears, ligament damage, and joint irritation similarly as pain from the ligament. Other than drugs, treatment will be facilitated to keep up the quality and extent of development of the hip. Correspondingly, likewise, with any ailment or harm, the goal is to reestablish the patient to their average level of limit. A gathering approach, including the social protection capable, physical counsel, or chiropractic care provider, may be considered.

Distress frequently might be made to do with over-the-counter pain meds. Acetaminophen, ibuprofen, and naproxen all might be utilized. Although these medications don't require relief has its very own potential for symptoms if basic ailments are available.

Knee Pain

Pain or discomfort in the knee can emerge from numerous sources. Knee pain can even originate from problems in the hip. Meniscus and ligament aggravation around the knee can cause pain. Pain can also emerge from kneecap (patella) issues or malt racking. Bracing the muscles around your knee will make it progressively enduring.

On the off chance that you are physically dynamic at practice or a game, you may need activities to address development designs that might influence your knees and to build up an excellent method during your sport or action. Exercises to improve your adaptability and equalization additionally are significant.

Ankle and Foot Pain

Pain from the lower leg can happen from lower leg sprains or ligament disturbance around the lower leg. Agony can likewise occur from ligament wounds around the lower leg and now and again, tendons and ligament just as lower leg joint inflammation can cause pain. Agony in the curve of the foot is frequently plantar fasciitis.

The medical procedure is now and then prescribed to improve the structure of your feet. If different medications haven't helped, medical procedure might be recommended to:

- Right valgus heel or mallet toes expel a neuroma or rheumatoid knob expel some portion of the bone from a bunion and reshape your toes soothe the pain.

- Joint substitutions for the lower leg and foot aren't yet as fruitful as substitution knees and hips. Most foot medical procedure is planned for rectifying the places of the joints by resetting the bones or combining the joint in the amended position.

What are the outcomes of those treatments?

An accumulation of activities, for example, quality preparing, heart fortifying action, degree of advancement and judo, can help with both pain and physical breaking point in knee osteoarthritis (OA). Reinforcing can, in the same way, help with hip OA pain. Water-based activities may improve work in the knee and hip joints, yet offer minor inclinations for pain.

Right when the biomechanics of the hip and knee joint are balanced or mishandled, the joint ends up being progressively disposed to the movements of osteoarthritis. Anatomical varieties in hip morphology in the people have been associated with the improvement of osteoarthritis.

How effective is treating tarsal tunnel syndrome with the medical procedure?

A large portion of people utilize their feet pretty much every moment of the day without the slightest hesitation. In any case, on the off chance that you have tarsal passage disorder, the pain, deadness, and shivering in your fingers stand out enough to be noticed. Tarsal tunnel syndrome is a compression or squeezing, on the posterior tibial nerve that produces symptoms anywhere along the path of the nerve running from the inside of the ankle into the foot. This syndrome is precisely similar to carpal tunnel syndrome, which occurs in the wrist. Medications like twist props and corticosteroids can help; however, in increasingly severe cases, you may require medical procedure.

Tarsal entry issue is achieved by weight on your center nerve. Exactly when the nerve encounters your foot, it experiences the tarsal section - a secure way that is made of bone and ligament. If you get any swelling in your feet, that section gets squashed and crushes your center nerve. That, in this manner, causes your appearances.

A counterfeit knee doesn't react to your resistant framework as your knee would. So if microorganisms get around your fake knee, it might duplicate and cause contamination.

What variables might be available that keep a patient from being not able to have a joint Replacement. (Age, diabetes, bone thickness, COPD, cardiovascular illnesses .and so forth)?

Shockingly, a couple of individuals will not be able to have a joint substitution, notwithstanding the way that their joint agony is dreadful. This may be because:

- Their thigh muscles (quadriceps) are slight and will, in all probability, is not able to assist their new knee joint.

- There are significant or suffering open injuries (ulcers) in the skin underneath the knee, extending the threat of bullying.

- Age factor: The average age of having a joint replacement in the United States is right around 65 years old. Generally, surgeons consider anyone under the age of 50 to be 'young' to have a joint replacement. Age more than 65years has a risk of surgery failure because of arthritis.

- Diabetes: Diabetes shows various effects on joint replacement surgery as it increases the risk of several complications including, higher risk of infection, higher risk of wound healing problem, higher risk of medical complications, etc.

- Bone thickness: the bone quality around the joint may affect the safety of prosthetic implantation and consequently, satisfaction with the surgical outcomes.

What is the risk of infection, amputation, death from total knee or hip replacement surgery?

Everyone who has a knee replaced is at risk for a deep infection. Most infections occur in the first two years after surgery. Still, you're at risk for a disease as long as you have the joint.

The implant itself puts you at risk for infection because bacteria can attach to it. An artificial knee doesn't respond to your immune system as your knee would. So if bacteria get around your artificial knee, it may multiply and cause an infection.

Plus, an infection anywhere in your body can travel to your knee. A common way bacteria gets into your body is through a break or wound in your skin, even a tiny one. Bacteria also often get in your body during major dental surgery. For example, your risk of infection increases when you have a tooth pulled or a root canal.

What is the risk of infection, amputation, death from total knee or hip replacement surgery?

Death in 90 days after hip substitution is very uncommon. A recent report in The Journal of Bone and Joint Surgery, American Edition, found that coronary illness was the primary source of death inside 90 days of medical procedure. They likewise observed an expansion in stomach related framework related passing.

The 30-day death rate for an absolute knee substitution (TKR) is around 1 out of 400, or 0.25 percent. That implies that 99.75 percent of the individuals who experience this medical procedure endure the treatment. Analysts indicated just about 2,500 individuals who had a TKR over a 10-year range.

After a knee substitution, your knee will feel warm and look red and swollen for around a few months. Firmness and soreness usually keep going three to a half year before continuously dying down. You'll have full recuperation around 12-year and a half after your medical procedure.

What is the risk of clots or complications?

Sitting in a vehicle, transport, or plane for extensive periods

When you travel for quite a while, you may sit still for the vast majority of the voyage, which can raise your danger of blood clumps, as indicated by the CDC. The more you're still, the more noteworthy your danger of building up coagulation.

The CDC takes note of that moving your legs regularly and strolling around each a few hours can help bring down your danger of creating DVT while voyaging. You can even add on specific activities, such as expanding your legs out and flexing your lower legs or inquire as to whether they have particular proposals for how to bring down your hazard.

If you realize you have other DVT hazard factors, you might need to chat with your primary care physician before setting out on a long trip. They may recommend you use anticoagulants, wear pressure leggings to shield blood from pooling in your legs, or find a way to maintain a strategic distance from blood clumps.

Smoking

Illuminating harms an entire host of your body's procedures, and your circulatory framework is no particular case. Smoking can hurt the coating of your veins and furthermore make it more probable that platelets in your blood will stick together, the two of which can add to excessive blood thickening, as indicated by the American Heart Association. In any case, stopping smoking is generally more complicated than one might expect. Here are seven hints to kick you off, and you can usually approach your primary care physician for increasingly explicit guidance. "It's unquestionably worth stopping smoking for your general wellbeing," Dr. Evans says.

Being more seasoned

While individuals of all ages can get blood coagulation, the Mayo Clinic records being more seasoned than 60 as one of the significant hazard factors for creating DVT (deep vein thrombosis). The explanations behind this aren't surely known, Dr. Evans says. Be that as it may, it might just be that, as you get more established, you're bound to create other wellbeing conditions or ailments that expansion your danger of creating DVT, similar to malignant growth, Dr. Fisher says. It likewise may be that your blood can clot as you get more established, he says. In any case, there's a great deal of vulnerability around this one.

"Indeed, even solid old patients are at more danger of clusters than their more youthful partners," Dr. Evans says. "There is something in particular about the science of maturing that expands coagulating potential."

Having a thickening issue

Some draining issue, similar to hemophilia and idiopathic thrombocytopenic purpura (ITP), influence your blood not to cluster enough. Others, similar to Factor V Leiden, fall on the contrary side of the range. These can make your blood hypercoagulable, which means it clumps way too effectively. While the side effects shift by condition, on the off chance that they do in certainty lead to blood coagulation or aspiratory embolism, you can expect typical manifestations like warmth, delicacy, redness, the brevity of pain, a quick heartbeat, and chest pain.

What limitation exists post-surgery?

- Do not evacuate the dressings.

- Try not to sit in the same position for more than 45 to 60 minutes at a time.

- DO NOT bend, squat, or reach for anything while you are showering

- When you are going upstairs, step first with your leg that did NOT have surgery.

- When you are going downstairs, step first with your leg that DID have surgery.

- Use your crutches or walker until your provider tells you it is OK to stop, which is often around 4 to 6 weeks after surgery. Use a cane only when your provider tells you it is OK.

- In general, avoid sports that require jerking, twisting, pulling, or running.

- DO NOT lift or carry more than 20 pounds (9 kilograms). This will place too much stress on your new knee.

- Take the mitigating and anti-microbial drugs as endorsed.

- Do not take Motrin or ibuprofen-like prescriptions.

- Bruising and Swelling would be expected.

- Numbness may continue during this period.

- The itching sensation could be an indication that you are oversensitive to something on foot.

- Mild hurt or throbbing can happen and is generally connected with a lot of standing or strolling.

How often does a joint replacement occur in the USA?

Substitution arthroplasty or joint substitution medical procedure is a technique of orthopedic medical procedure where a ligament or broken joint surface is supplanted with an orthopedic prosthesis. Joint substitution is considered as a treatment when less-intrusive treatments don't ease severe joint pain or brokenness. It is a type of arthroplasty and is frequently demonstrated from different joint illnesses, including osteoarthritis and rheumatoid joint pain. Every year, over 600,000 knee replacement surgeries are carried out in the United States.

What is the typical rehab and downtime required?

Exercise-based recuperation is a significant piece of the mending procedure and is fundamental on the off chance that you intend to diminish your knee substitution recuperation time. A physiotherapist will show you useful joint activities and will work with you to draft a short-and long haul recuperation activity plan. On account of the littler cut, insignificantly intrusive knee substitution recuperation time might be shorter than the mending time related with a conventional knee substitution system.

Hip bone Rehab:

- Get in a sound exercise schedule.

- Most hip substitution patients can stroll around the same time or following day of medical procedure; most can continue routine exercises inside the initial 3 to about a month and a half of their complete hip substitution recuperation.

- Focus on eating routine and weight.

- Overabundance weight can put pressure on your new hip prosthesis and increment wear and the danger of confusion.

Most patients can care for themselves and resume normal daily activities within six weeks and drive within 3 to 6 weeks. It may take 4 to 6 months or up to an entire year to fully recover and realize the total benefits of knee replacement surgery.

How often are steroids used to treat extremities?

Surgeons, on the whole, don't like you to have a steroid injection into a joint they are likely to operate on in the near (some say up to six months) future. Week by week dosages of glucocorticoid steroids, for example, prednisone, help speed recuperation in muscle wounds, reports another Northwestern Medicine to concentrate distributed in the Journal of Clinical Investigation and the week by week steroids likewise fixed muscles harmed by robust dystrophy.

One of the severe issues of utilizing steroids, for example, prednisone is they cause muscle squandering and shortcoming when taken long haul. This is a noteworthy issue for individuals who take steroids for some interminable conditions, and can regularly bring about patients halting steroid medications.

How successful are steroids?

Infusing steroids close to the tarsal passage is a typical treatment. Steroids decrease swelling in the connective tissue, which diminishes the weight on the median nerve. The advantages of steroid infusions have been tried in a few examinations

They found that indications improved in numerous individuals within two months of treatment:

- Complete recovery occurred in around 30 out of 100 individuals.

- Indications improved after steroids were infused in approximately 75 out of 100 individuals.

What is the risk of using steroids over time?

A few steroids can be unfathomably destructive to the individuals who take them. There is a wide array of serious side effects associated with abuse of steroids. Steroid use can alter the normal hormonal production in the body. Most side effects can be reversed if the drugs are stopped, but some, such as a deepened voice in women may persist. Data on long-term side effects primarily come from case reports and not from well-controlled, long-term epidemiological studies, which might be more reliable. Major negative effects include kidney, liver and heart diseases. In addition, prolonged use of steroids can lead to physiological and psychological addiction.

What is the occurrence of repeat procedures in the knee and hip bone?

It's critical to take note of that a modification knee substitution doesn't give a similar life expectancy as the underlying substitution (typically around ten years as opposed to 20). The gathered injury, scar tissue, and mechanical breakdown of segments lead to reduced execution. Amendments are likewise increasingly defenseless to intricacies.

A correction system is ordinarily more intricate than the first knee substitution medical procedure because the specialist must expel the first embed, which would have developed into the current bone. Also, when the specialist expels the prosthesis, there is less bone remaining. In certain occurrences, a bone joins transplanting a bit of bone transplanted from another piece of the body or a contributor may be required to help the new prosthesis. A bone join includes support and energizes new bone development.

Be that as it may, the technique requires extra preoperative arranging, particular devices, and more prominent careful aptitude. The medical procedure takes more time to perform than an essential introductory knee substitution.

What is the life expectancy after an older adult has a hip replacement Surgery?

Numerous conditions lead to degeneration of the hip joint and the possible requirement for hip substitution. All out hip substitution medical procedure keeps on being the treatment of decision for weakening essential osteoarthritis, the significant sign for 70% of hip tasks. Different indications include hip dysplasia with or without separation, hip crack, rheumatoid joint pain, and avascular putrefaction. The beneficial outcome that total hip substitution medical procedure has on the personal satisfaction of patients is colossal and settled. Absolute hip substitution medical procedure is, nonetheless, trying for both the specialist and the patient. Staying up with the latest with advancements in this specific territory of the orthopedic medical system is the way to giving patients the best guidance and accomplishing the best outcomes for them.

Effectiveness of treating neuropathy in hands and feet with medication? Risks and benefits? I.e.: (gabapentin)

Gabapentin at parts of 1800 mg to 3600 mg step by step (1200 mg to 3600 mg gabapentin encarbil) can give extraordinary degrees of assistance with inconvenience to specific people with post-therapeutic neuralgia and periphery diabetic neuropathy. Evidence for various types of neuropathic anguish is incredibly confined. The consequence of in any occasion half pain power reduction is seen as an accommodating aftereffect of treatment by patients, and the achievement of this degree of alleviation from distress is connected with noteworthy beneficial effects on rest impedance, weariness, and despairing, similarly as close to home fulfillment, limit, and work. Around 3 or 4 out of 10 individuals achieved this degree of help from inconvenience with gabapentin, differentiated and 1 or 2 out of 10 for phony treatment. Over part of those treated with gabapentin won't have invaluable assistance with uneasiness anyway may experience opposing events.

CHAPTER: 17

MENISCUS TEAR AND KNEE DEGENERATION

Meniscus Tears

We often hear the following term in sports injuries called Meniscus Tears or Meniscal Tear? What are they, how do they happen, how do we know that we have a Meniscus Tear, and most importantly how do we fix them? These are all very important questions and thoughts when one is presented with a Meniscus Tear. The meniscus is primarily considered a cartilage that is used as a protective "layer" to protect your knee and your knee joints. This cartilage is also used to allow for one's body weight to consume the energy impact that is spread on one's knee. There are generally two types of Meniscus that surround the knee and knee joints. The first is called the Medial Meniscus which consumes the inner part of one's knee, and the other is called the Lateral Meniscus, and that is consumed by the outer portion of one's knee.

What is Meniscus Tear?

The meniscus is a rubbery, C-shaped disc that supports and cushions the knee. Injury to this part of the knee is common. There are two menisci in each knee. One is at the outer or lateral side of the knee, and the other is at the inner, or medial, side. These structures keep the knee steady by allowing for a balance of weight across the knee. If one of these menisci is torn, the knee does not function properly, and the torn meniscus can scuff and damage the surfaces of the knee resulting in arthritis.

Meniscus tears occur on the C-shaped disc that supports and cushions the knee. When this structure is damaged or torn, there may be pain, swelling, stiffness, and limited range of motion. Twisting or turning incorrectly can bring on a meniscus tear or injury. Knee arthroscopy is a safe procedure the orthopedic specialist may perform to repair a meniscus tear and diagnose the extent of the injury to the knee.

Meniscus Tears happen frequently, and they are mostly seen among athletes or those who participate in contact sports. Sports which include football, basketball, tennis, and soccer are the most common types of activity where Meniscus Tears are experienced. Although a variety of factors can contribute to such an injury, it most frequently occurs when the knee is planted on the ground and is then twisted in a violent or unorthodox fashion.

It will also help to understand that meniscus tear has three levels, which include the following:

1. Mild Tear where you will experience slight pain and a little swelling of the knee

2. Moderate Tear where pain increases and swelling becomes obvious. Here, you may find it difficult to move your knees and may restrict some activities such as squatting or walking.

3. Severe Tear where pain and swelling become almost unbearable. Your movement is restrained, and you may even find it hard to stand up as your knees can give way suddenly at any time.

What are the Symptoms of a Meniscus Tear?

Although people may experience a variety of different symptoms associated with tearing their Meniscus cartilage. The most common complaint from individuals include pain and swelling around the knee area. The knee will usually be sensitive to touch, and the range of motion can be limited to certain people. In addition, some people may experience sounds when extending their knee or when trying to move their knee outwards. These sounds have been reported as clicking or cracking sounds, and those can sometimes be attributed to the torn Meniscal cartilage.

The symptoms associated with meniscus tears vary greatly depending on the severity. Minor tears may result in slight pain and swelling. If there are no mechanical symptoms, such as catching or locking, these tears may resolve on their own in around 2 or 3 weeks. More moderate tears can lead to pain at the side and back of the knee. The swelling of a moderate tear slowly gets worse over a 2 or 3 day period. The knee will feel stiff with this type of injury, and there will be limitations to how far the knee can be bent. The symptoms may go away after a week or two but can come back anytime there is re-injury or overuse of the knee. The pain of a moderate tear could go on for years if the tear is not treated properly.

The third type of tear is a severe tear. With these, pieces of the meniscus are torn and can displace into the joint space. This will make the knee pop, catch or lock without notice. It will be difficult to straighten the knee as well. The knee may be described as "wobbly" and give way without any warning. Most people who suffer a severe tear have pain, swelling and stiffness immediately following the injury and it gets worse over the next few days.

Generally, people with torn meniscus feel pain while walking or straightening the knee. Other common signs of a torn meniscus include a swelling and stiffness in and around the knee. These symptoms may become worse if the torn meniscus fragments get caught in the knee joint. This may lead to catching sensations in the knee. If a large enough piece of meniscus becomes loose and lodges between the thigh bone and tibia, this may cause your knee to slip or lock.

How common is Meniscus Tear in the United States?

The meniscus is a piece of cartilage that provides a cushion between your femur (thighbone) and tibia (shinbone). There are two menisci in each knee joint. They can be damaged or torn during activities that put pressure on or rotate the knee joint. Taking a hard tackle on the football field or a sudden pivot on the basketball court can result in a meniscus tear. You don't have to be an athlete to get a meniscus tear, though. Simply getting up too quickly from a squatting position can also cause a meniscal tear. According to Boston Children's Hospital, more than 500,000 meniscal tears take place in the United States each year. Also, there has been an increased number of isolated meniscus repairs being performed in the US over the past 7 years without a concomitant increase in meniscectomies over the same time frame.

Meniscus surgeries are the most common arthroscopic surgery in the United States, with roughly one million procedures annually. The Arthroscopic surgery is a minimally invasive surgical procedure performed by an orthopedic surgeon in which a damaged joint is treated, through small incisions with specialized tools, under the guidance of a tiny camera called an arthroscope.

What causes Meniscus Tear?

A tear of a meniscus is a rupturing of one or more of the fibrocartilage strips in the knee called menisci. When doctors and patients refer to "torn cartilage" in the knee, they actually may be referring to an injury to a meniscus at the top of one of the tibiae. Menisci can be torn during innocuous activities such as walking or squatting. They can also be torn by traumatic force encountered in sports or other forms of physical exertion. The traumatic action is most often a twisting movement at the knee while the leg is bent.

Common causes of a meniscus tear include:

1. Meniscus tears can happen when a person changes direction suddenly while running. Although they're more common in athletes who play contact sports, meniscus tears can happen to runners. In runners, the meniscus is often injured by a twisting motion or a blow to the side of the knee. Older athletes are more at risk since the meniscus weakens with age. Runners more commonly injure the medial meniscus (central meniscus attached to the tibia or shinbone) rather than the lateral meniscus (on the side of the knee).

2. A torn meniscus can result from any activity that causes you to forcefully twist or rotate your knees, such as aggressive pivoting or sudden stops and turns. Even kneeling, deep squatting or lifting something heavy can sometimes lead to a torn meniscus. In older adults, degenerative changes of the knee can contribute to a torn meniscus with little or no trauma.

3. Tears can lead to pain and/or swelling of the knee joint. Especially acute injuries (typically in younger, more active patients) can lead to displaced tears which can cause mechanical symptoms such as clicking, catching, or locking during motion of the knee joint. The joint will be in pain when in use, but when there is no load, the pain goes away.

4. Rapid stepping or squatting on an uneven surface can cause a

disproportionate force on the knees, leading to tears or ruptures of the meniscus. This movement might occur while trail running in cross country, running football drills, or falling awkwardly in lacrosse.

5. Also, in older adults, the meniscus can be damaged following prolonged 'wear and tear' called a degenerative tear. People with a degenerative joint condition, or who engage in activity or professions that involve a lot of squatting up and down, are susceptible to developing a meniscal tear. Degenerative conditions, such as knee osteoarthritis, can cause tears in either of the menisci over time. This sort of condition weakens the cartilage of the meniscus, allowing it to be torn with greater ease.

6. Twisting or turning quickly can lead to a meniscus tear. Often, the foot is planted while the knee is bent. These types of tears occur when the person is lifting something heavy or playing sports. As people get older, the likelihood of meniscus wear and tear increases. Unexpected, quick force can lead the knee joint to flex too far back and tear the meniscus. For example, colliding with the leg of another basketball player while coming down from a rebound might cause this.

How is a Meniscus Tear Diagnosed?

Before the proper treatment of a meniscus tear can be recommended by a physician, a proper diagnosis must be made and confirmed. The symptoms of a meniscus tear include pain and swelling of the knee joint. These symptoms are also common in cases of arthritis and ligament and/or tendon tears. A physical examination in the clinical setting, as well as diagnostic imaging, will be the first step in determining if a meniscal tear is present.

For patients that have some metal implants, pacemakers, or spinal cord or nerve stimulators, etc., a CT scan is the next best diagnostic imaging test that can be performed. Once a positive clinical diagnosis is made, and the diagnostic images confirm the clinical findings, a treatment can be recommended. Most of the time, the orthopedic specialist inquires with the patient regarding past injuries and accidents. The doctor will also perform a physical examination to help find out if the meniscus is torn and causes pain. Testing may involve X-Rays and/or an MRI so the doctor can see if the meniscus is torn and how severe the injury is.

How is Meniscus Tear treated?

Treatment for meniscus tears depends on the size and location of the tear. Other factors which influence treatment include age, activity level, and related injuries. The outer portion of the meniscus often referred to as the "red zone," has a good blood supply and can sometimes heal on its own if the tear is small. In contrast, the inner two-thirds of the meniscus, known as the "white zone," does not have a good blood supply. Tears in this region will not heal on their own as this area lacks blood vessels to bring in healing nutrients.

The degree of aggressiveness when approaching the treatment options is based on the extensiveness of the meniscus tear. Meniscus tears are classified based on the anatomical region of the meniscus that is affected and how deep into the tissue the tear occurs. Medial meniscal tears occur on the inside of the knee. Lateral meniscus tears occur on the outside of the knee. Horizontal tears occur in the front part of the knee and run parallel with the tibial plateau (knee end of the tibia).

Radial tears occur at center of the "C" shaped structure and go across the middle dividing the meniscus. Oblique or meniscal flap tears can occur at any part of the meniscus but are most likely to be found in the ends of the "C" shaped structure. Complex or degenerative tears include more than one tear and are usually gradual over time as opposed to a specific event causing an acute tear.

There are several factors based on which a doctor will determine which treatment will work best for your torn meniscus. These factors include the location of the tear, the pattern of the tear, the extent and size of the tear. Your age, pain level, and activity level may also affect your treatment options.

However, the following are treatment options for a meniscus tear:

Conservative Management

In almost all cases of a meniscus tear conservative management (non-operative) is the first treatment option. This treatment involves steroid knee injections to reduce inflammation and swelling, physical therapy for six to nine weeks, and wearing a knee brace in everyday life to help take some of the load off of the joint while the body has a chance to repair the tear on its own. Patients that have symptomatic meniscus tears can expect a 50% chance of full resolution of pain and symptoms with conservative treatment.

The steroid injections reduce the inflammation and swelling of the knee joint. Some of the pain can be reduced from these injections as well. This can allow for more productive physical therapy appointments. The physical therapy can assist with realigning the body mechanics with respect to movement. This will also stop the knee joint from freezing up and will reduce soreness. Physical Therapy is administered by a licensed Physical Therapist. A list of exercises is performed by the patient concentrating on stretching and moving the knee joint in a controlled fashion under the supervision of the physical therapist.

Surgical Treatment

Patients that fail to respond to conservative treatment must consider surgical options to pursue the achievement of a reduction in pain and symptoms associated with a meniscal tear. The majorities of tears that need this next step are usually advanced in the severity of the tear or have an abundance of scar tissue around the tear that has prevented the proper collagen tissue from being deposited. State of the art standards of care now includes arthroscopic surgical intervention options. The goal of all surgical options is to relieve pain and symptoms associated with the meniscal tear. Choosing the correct surgical option is based on the severity and location of the meniscus tear.

Arthroscopic Surgery

Advances in arthroscopic procedures have allowed the meniscus to be surgically repaired by the use of a camera and endoscopic surgical instrumentation. These surgeries are typically performed outpatient at a surgery center. The most common surgery is an arthroscopic meniscal "shaving" technique. A scope is inserted into the knee joint, and then the joint is filled with a saline solution. The scope is connected to an intra-operative television monitor allowing the surgeon to view the inside of the knee joint. Next, a shaver is inserted into the knee to shave off scar tissue and the jagged edges of the tear. Again this will allow the body to heal the tear with collagen.

Nonsurgical Treatment

If your tear is small and on the outer edge of the meniscus, it may not require surgical repair. As long as your symptoms do not persist and your knee is stable, nonsurgical treatment may be all you need. Common nonsurgical treatments for meniscus tears include:

RICE: As the first line of treatment, RICE consists of (1) Resting, (2) Icing at regular intervals, (3) Compressing the knee with a compression wrap, and (4) Elevating the injured knee. This initial approach will help keep the swelling at bay in the first few hours and days following the injury.

Anti-inflammatory medication: A type of non-steroidal anti-inflammatory medication (NSAID), such as ibuprofen (E.g., Advil), may be given to reduce swelling shortly after the injury.

Physical therapy: Prescribed physical therapy is often recommended after the injury, after surgery, or both. The goals of physical therapy are usually to control pain and swelling, help restore the normal range of motion to the knee, improve strength in the muscles that support the knee.

Electrical stimulation: Neuromuscular electrical stimulation of the muscles in the knee may be used with the goal of strengthening the meniscus and surrounding tissues.

Injections: Corticosteroid injections into the knee joint may be used in order to relieve pain or inflammation in the soft tissue of the knee.

What Are Some Of The Side Effects Associated With The Treatment Of Meniscus Tear?

There may be some complications associated with surgery for meniscal tears, including unforeseen complications with anesthesia, such as respiratory or cardiac malfunction. Infections may result from surgery, in addition to the injury of the nerves and blood vessels, fracture, weakness, stiffness or instability of the joint, pain, inability to repair the meniscus, repeated rupture of the meniscus, or the need for additional surgeries.

Patients should be made aware that not all meniscal tears are repairable. The cartilage in the knee may have simply worn away over time, preventing the surgeon from repairing the remaining cartilage with sutures. In these cases, the surgeon will remove all the torn cartilage and repair any other problems in the knee.

Surgical procedures and risks associated with meniscal surgery will depend on the patient's condition and his or her individual needs. Patients should keep in mind that their age does play an important role in the success of the procedure. Repairs tend to be most effective for people under the age of 30 who have the procedure done within the first two months after injury. For people over 30, the likelihood of success of surgery diminishes because the meniscal tissue begins to deteriorate and weaken with age naturally.

Knee Degeneration What is Knee Degeneration?

Degenerative knee disease, also known as osteoarthritis is due to the loss of cartilage within your joints. Degenerative joint disease is a progressive disorder that attacks the body's cartilage, which is the hard tissue that covers up the end of bones and meets the joints, allowing bones to move.

Degenerative joint disease is believed to be the most common form of arthritis there is by far and the primary cause of joint pain in adults, usually affecting older people and slowly getting worse as they continue to age.

The terms degenerative joint disease, degenerative arthritis, and osteoarthritis are often used interchangeably. Both are essentially the same type of disorder that results in cartilage (tissue between your bones) wearing down over time and causing a lot of bone and joint pain in the process. Osteoarthritis is degenerative in nature because it worsens as time goes on, and unfortunately there isn't a known "cure" at this time to stop it from progressing or to reverse the damage already done.

Arthritis has been known to inflame the knee joint or even cause malformations. But you may also be experiencing slight pinches or jolts of pains as you climb a stairway or feel some grinding now and then. We know that degeneration of the knee joint is a chronic disease that causes pain and in many cases can incapacitate, so much so that often surgery for a knee replacement is recommended.

How common is Knee Degeneration in the United States?

The prevalence of knee arthritis among people in the United States has doubled since the start of World War II. Osteoarthritis (OA) is the most prevalent joint disease and a leading source of chronic pain and disability in the United States and other developed nations. Knee OA accounts for more than 80% of the disease's total burden and affects at least 20% of American adults aged 45 and older. Substantial evidence indicates that knee OA is proximately caused by the breakdown of joint tissues from mechanical loading and inflammation, but the deeper underlying causes of knee OA's high prevalence remain unclear and poorly tested, hindering efforts to prevent and treat the disease.

Two recent public health trends, however, are commonly assumed to be dominant factors. First, because knee OA's prevalence increases with age, the rise in life expectancy in the United States since the early 20th century is thought to have led to high knee OA levels among the elderly, with the presumption that, as people age, their senescing joint tissues accumulate more wear and tear from loading. Second, high body mass index (BMI) has become epidemic in the United States in recent decades and is a well-known risk factor for knee OA, probably because of the combined effects of joint overloading and adiposity-induced inflammation. Whether increases in longevity and BMI are responsible for current knee OA levels has never been tested, but this assumption has led many to view the disease's high prevalence as effectively unpreventable, since aging is untreatable, and the high BMI epidemic is intractable.

Today, almost 20% of people in the United States over 45 years old suffer from knee osteoarthritis, in which joint cartilage breaks down; the odds of developing it climb as we get older. Scientists have long suspected that number has risen in recent generations. Because most Americans are living significantly longer than their grandparents, researchers have speculated that the graying population could be one culprit.

Projecting new and advanced cases of knee OA among persons aged 60–64 years over the next decade creates a benchmark that can be used to evaluate population-based benefits of future disease-modifying OA drugs that are currently undergoing testing at various stages.

What Causes Knee Degeneration?

Arthritis is the leading cause of knee joint degeneration. In many cases, genetics or hereditary diseases are to blame for the condition and may include obesity or excess weight that puts stress on the joint. There are rare occasions where the degeneration does not appear to have any origin. People may experience a slight alteration of their joint's cartilage cells, or malformation of muscles or subchondral bone alignment which causes an undesirable alignment and resistance in the joint as well as affecting the elasticity of the cartilage causes cartilage thinning and deterioration.

The degenerative joint disease causes are typically wear and tear injuries that occur over time. In fact, advanced age is a major risk factor of degenerative joint disease, and it is rare for anyone over the age of 70 to be unaffected in some way by this progressive disorder.

Though degenerative joint disease, also known as osteoarthritis, can come on as a consequence of everyday life, its onset can be sped up by certain factors, which include the following.

- Trauma due to sports

- Trauma from work-related activities or injuries

- Repetitive motions of a joint for a long time

- Infection in a joint

- Excess weight, which puts pressure on the weight-bearing joints.

Degenerative joint disease is common in the weight-bearing joints (spine, hips, knees, ankles, feet, and toes) but can also occur in the non-weight bearing joints (shoulders, elbows, wrists, hands, and fingers).

How is Knee Degeneration Treated?

The effective treatment and management program focuses on the pain and mechanical components of the degenerative knee disease.

Pain control and management is done by providing appropriate intervention to treat both local pain and systemic pain. Over the counter pain, medication and non-steroidal anti-inflammatory medications are typically recommended to manage the systemic pain whereas cryotherapy, intra-articular cortisone injections, and electrical stimulation can be done to control the local pain. Always speak to your physician regarding the use of any medication.

The mechanical component of the treatment regimen involves a comprehensive weight reducing program. Being overweight puts excessive strain on the knees, and even if this was not the direct cause of the condition, it can aggravate the knee and cause it to deteriorate even faster. Contrary to popular misconception, exercising can actually be useful if you have degenerative knee disease. Not only does it help keep your weight down, but it also helps keep the knee flexible. The recommended activities will typically be low impact such as swimming.

Other common home remedies for degenerative joint disease are:

- OTC (over-the-counter) drugs like acetaminophen (Tylenol) are the first remedy tried by most osteoarthritis sufferers. Aspirin will have similar pain-relieving effects but may be harder on your stomach

- NSAIDS (Nonsteroidal anti-inflammatory drugs) like ibuprofen and naproxen can provide some relief from pain and are commonly thought of as a step up from Tylenol or Aspirin. Talk with your doctor if you feel a need for regular use of these pain relievers.

- OTC glucosamine and chondroitin formulas have mixed results, but some claim good results with their regular use.

- There are a number of pain-relieving lotions and creams. Try Capsaicin (Zostrix), this may feel unusual at first but has proven to be helpful for the temporary relief of degenerative joint disease.

- Hot or cold packs may provide temporary relief. Hot packs can warm the joint and aid in pain-free movement. Cold packs help reduce swelling and pain that may occur following exercise.

- Allow sufficient time to rest the affected joint and if repetitive movements aggravate the symptoms, take a step to change your routine.

- You do not want to avoid exercise because it helps to keep your joints mobile. However, you may need to shift your exercise routine to exercises that do not stress your joints. Swimming and water activities are non-weight bearing exercises. You can also walk instead of a jog to put knees under less stress.

- Alternative treatments like acupuncture and massage may provide you with relief. If your pain, swelling, and stiffness is getting worse or interfering with your daily life, you should consult your doctor.

What Are Some Of The Side Effects Associated With The Treatment Of Knee Degeneration?

Osteoarthritis (OA) a common disease of the aged population and one of the leading causes of disability. The incidence of knee OA is rising by increasing the average age of the general population. Age, weight, trauma to joint due to repetition movements, in particular, squatting and kneeling are common risk factors of knee OA.

Many people have no adverse effects after a steroid injection besides a little pain or tingling where the injection was made. However, corticosteroids can cause dangerous side effects for some people, especially when taken too often.

Also, Viscosupplementation is considered a safe procedure, but like any medical procedure, it does carry some risks and side effects. Patients should talk to their doctors about these potential risks and complications, which are described below.

Patients who undergo viscosupplementation may have mild discomfort immediately after the procedure. Typical side effects at the injection site include Localized swelling, Skin warmth and redness, Soreness, and Joint stiffness.

CHAPTER: 18

ANTERIOR CRUCIATE INJURIES

What is an Anterior Cruciate Ligament Tear?

The Anterior Cruciate Ligament (ACL) is one of a pair of cruciate ligaments (the other being the posterior cruciate ligament) in the human knee. An anterior cruciate ligament injury is the over-stretching or tearing of the anterior cruciate ligament (ACL) in the knee. A tear may be partial or complete. The anterior cruciate ligament is a vital ligament inside the knee joint for providing stability of the knee. It can get injured in sport or as a consequence of an accident.

In sport, it is usually due to a non-contact rotational injury at the knee, and the player is unable to continue the game. The two ligaments are also called cruciform ligaments, as they are arranged in a crossed formation. In the quadruped stifle joint (analogous to the knee), based on its anatomical position, it is also referred to as the cranial cruciate ligament. The anterior cruciate ligament is one of the four main ligaments of the knee, providing 85% of the restraining force to anterior tibial displacement at 30 degrees and 90 degrees of knee flexion.

The ACL is the most commonly injured ligament in the knee. People often tear the ACL by changing direction rapidly, slowing down from running, or landing from a jump. When you twist your knee or fall on it, you can tear this stabilizing ligament that connects your thighbone to your shinbone. When the ACL tears, it unravels like a braided rope and does not heal on its own. Once the ACL is torn, the knee usually becomes unstable. Females, for many different reasons, are more likely to injure their ACL than males. Injuries to the ACL can occur in a number of situations, including sports, and can be quite severe, requiring surgery.

How Common is Anterior Cruciate Ligament Tears in the United States?

The anterior cruciate ligament (ACL) is the most frequently injured ligament in the knee for which surgery is performed. United States national estimates of ACL reconstruction vary widely. The PCL and anterior cruciate ligament (ACL) limit the motion of the tibia backward and forward, respectively. The lateral collateral ligament (on the outside of the knee) and the medial collateral ligament (on the inside of the knee) limit side-to-side knee motion.

About 200,000 people are affected per year in the United States. In some sports, females have a higher risk of an ACL injury, while in others, both sexes are equally affected. Many people with a complete tear who do not receive surgery are unable to play sports and may develop osteoarthritis.

There are around 200,000 ACL tears each year in the United States, with over 100,000 ACL reconstruction surgeries per year. Over 95% of ACL reconstructions are performed in the outpatient setting. The most common procedures performed during ACL reconstruction are partial meniscectomy and chondroplasty.

The tears or ruptures of the anterior cruciate ligament (ACL) are a common type of knee injury, with approximately 200,000 reported annually in the United States. This type of injury frequently occurs in sports. ACL injuries commonly occur in the following instances:

- As a result of cutting, pivoting or single-leg landing, and without any external trauma

- Through a twisting force applied to the knee while the foot is planted on the ground, or upon landing on one foot

- From a direct trauma to the knee, usually, the outside of the knee, as may occur in many contact sports

What Causes Anterior Cruciate Ligament Tear?

People who suffer from a sudden anterior cruciate ligament (ACL) injury are typically aware when it happens. Most of the time, they feel or hear something like a pop sound and also the knee may give out, which can cause them to fall. With this kind of injury, the knee swells and the patient feels too much pain, and there is a loss of the capacity of the knee and the leg to move.

A typical ACL injury can cause minor or major tears of the ligament. There are many cases where there is a complete tear of the ligament. Also, some people suffer separation of the ligament from the lower or upper leg bone. There are times also when the ligament separates from a part of the bone or the rest of the bone. In case any of these take place, the lower bone of the leg gets dislocated forward on the upper bone, which then causes the knee to look as if it was buckling or giving out.

Once the anterior cruciate ligament tears, the blood vessels surrounding the torn ligament and blood penetrates the knee joint, which then causes swelling. In this case, even the doctor may find it hard to examine the injured knee because of the swelling.

The underlying mechanism often involves a rapid change in direction, sudden stop, landing after a jump, or direct contact to the knee. It is more common in athletes, particularly those who participate in alpine skiing, soccer, football, or basketball. Several studies have shown that female athletes have a higher incidence of ACL injury than male athletes in certain sports. It has been proposed that this is due to differences in physical conditioning, muscular strength, and neuromuscular control. Other suggested causes include differences in the pelvis and lower extremity (leg) alignment, increased looseness in ligaments, and the effects of estrogen on ligament properties.

ACL injury is most likely to occur in the following situations:

- Changing direction rapidly (also known as "cutting")

- Landing from a jump awkwardly

- Direct contact or collision to the knee (i.e., during a football tackle or a motor vehicle collision)

- Get hit very hard on the side of your knee, such as during a football tackle

- Overextend your knee joint

- Quickly stop moving and change direction while running, landing from a jump, or turning

- Slowing down while running

How is Anterior Cruciate Ligament Tears Treated?

There is likely to be immediate swelling and pain. This should be managed by RICE (Rest, Ice, Compression, and Elevation). It is important to consult an appropriate doctor as soon as possible. After a detailed history, the patient would have to be investigated with x-rays to rule out any bony injuries. If a soft-tissue injury is suspected (like ACL injury), an MRI may be necessary, to confirm the diagnosis and also to rule out other associated injuries like a meniscal injury or an injury to one of the other ligaments like PCL or Postero-lateral corner ligament complex. The treatment of anterior cruciate ligament tears can be nonsurgical treatment and surgical treatment.

Nonsurgical Treatment

In nonsurgical treatment, progressive physical therapy and rehabilitation can restore the knee to a condition close to its pre-injury state and educate the patient on how to prevent instability. This may be supplemented with the use of a hinged knee brace. However, many people who choose not to have surgery may experience secondary injury to the knee due to repetitive instability episodes.

Surgical treatment is usually advised in dealing with combined injuries (ACL tears in combination with other injuries in the knee). However, deciding against surgery is reasonable for select patients. Nonsurgical management of isolated ACL tears is likely to be successful or may be indicated in patients:

- With partial tears and no instability symptoms

- With complete tears and no symptoms of knee instability during low-demand sports who are willing to give up high-demand sports

- Who do light manual work or live sedentary lifestyles

- Whose growth plates are still open (children)

Surgical Treatment

ACL tears are not usually repaired using a suture to sew it back together, because repaired ACLs have generally been shown to fail over time.

Therefore, the torn ACL is generally replaced by a substitute graft made of tendon. The following are the procedure surgical treatment:

- Before any surgical treatment, the patient is usually sent to physical therapy. Patients who have a stiff, swollen knee lacking the full range of motion at the time of ACL surgery may have significant problems regaining motion after surgery. It usually takes three or more weeks from the time of injury to achieve full range of motion.

It is also recommended that some ligament injuries be braced and allowed to heal before ACL surgery.

- The patient, the surgeon, and the anesthesiologist select the anesthesia used for surgery. Patients may benefit from an anesthetic block of the nerves of the leg to decrease postoperative pain.

- The surgery usually begins with an examination of the patient's knee while the patient is relaxed due to the effects of anesthesia. This final examination is used to verify that the ACL is torn and also to check for looseness of other knee ligaments that may need to be repaired during surgery or addressed postoperatively.

- If the physical exam strongly suggests the ACL is torn, the selected tendon is harvested (for an autograft) or thawed (for an allograft), and the graft is prepared to the correct size for the patient. After the graft has been prepared, the surgeon places an arthroscope into the joint. Small (one-centimeter) incisions called portals are made in the front of the knee to insert the arthroscope and instruments, and the surgeon examines the condition of the knee. Meniscus and cartilage injuries are trimmed or repaired, and the torn ACL stump is then removed.

What Are Some Of The Side Effects Associated With The

Treatment Of Anterior Cruciate Ligament Tears?

Despite meticulous care, complications can occur following anterior cruciate ligament (ACL) reconstruction of the knee. The central third of the patella tendon is the most common graft used to reconstruct the ACL.

People who experience an ACL injury are at higher risk of developing knee osteoarthritis, in which joint cartilage deteriorates, and its smooth surface roughens. Arthritis may occur even if you have surgery to reconstruct the ligament. Multiple factors likely influence the risk of arthritis, such as the severity of the original injury, the presence of related injuries in the knee joint or the level of activity after treatment.

Also, because ACL reconstruction is a surgical procedure, it carries certain risks, which include the following:

- bleeding and blood clots

- continued knee pain

- disease transmission if the graft comes from a cadaver

- infection

- knee stiffness or weakness

- loss of range of motion

- improper healing if the graft is rejected by your immune system

What is PCL Posterior Cruciate Ligament Tear?

The knee is probably the most overused part of our body. We use it every single day without fail, and this increases the risk of injury. It is also one of the most flexible parts of our body with the other being our shoulder. To increase the flexibility of a joint, certain functions and strength will have to decrease, making it more prone to injuries.

Injuries to the PCL are not as common as injuries to the ACL. This is largely due to the higher tensile strength of the PCL as compared to the ACL. The main role of the PCL is to prevent posterior translation of the tibia on the femur. It also helps to provide rotation stability and axis control functions to the knee. Due to its less common nature, injuries to the PCL are usually not managed properly and thus, lead to poor clinical outcomes. Injuries to the PCL are often accompanied by injuries to the surrounding tissues.

The posterior cruciate ligament or PCL is a ligament located in the knee. The strong band of tissues that comprise the PCL serves to connect your tibia to your femur. More commonly people experience an injury to the anterior cruciate ligament (ACL), but it is also possible to experience a PCL injury or tear.

How Common is PCL Posterior Cruciate Ligament Tear in the United States?

Sports-related injuries, specifically the ligamentous injuries to the knee, are quite common these days, thanks to the dramatic increase in young population's interest and participation in sports. Each year in the United States, about 25,000 PCL injuries are diagnosed, roughly one-tenth the number of diagnosed ACL injuries. Fifty percent of PCL injuries occur in conjunction with other knee ligament injuries, while the other 50 percent occur alone and are referred to as isolated PCL injuries.

In modern times, PCL injuries during sports are inevitable when indulging in physically demanding or contact sports. PCL tears usually result from high force impacts, generally vehicular accidents or contact sports such as football, soccer, or hockey. PCL injuries also can occur in non-contact sports, such as gymnastics or skiing, but are much less common.

So much so that there is an altogether separate branch of medicine dedicated to the treatment of sports injuries and is called sports medicine. While minor wounds can heal in a few days or weeks, major ones may require surgical attention. However, just like any other surgery, surgical treatment of sports injuries may be expensive in the United States and other Western countries. But thanks to medical tourism, now these treatments can be obtained for cheap.

What Causes PCL Posterior Cruciate Ligament Tears?

There are a number of things that may cause a posterior cruciate ligament tear. Most commonly a PCL injury happens following some type of fall or other powerful strikes to the knee, particularly if the knee is bent during the incident. Certain sports may also have a higher likelihood of PCL tears, for example, soccer, skiing, and football.

PCL injuries span a range in severity from less severe to very severe. Typically during a physician's medical assessment for a PCL tear, during diagnosis, a physician may determine the grade of the injury, ranging from the most mild Grade 1 signifying a partial tearing of the PCL to the most severe Grade 4, when the PCL is torn along with other knee ligaments like for example the ACL.

The main cause of PCL injury is severe trauma to the knee joint. Often, other ligaments in the knee are affected as well. One cause specific to PCL injury is the hyperextension of the knee. This can occur during athletic movements like jumping. Athletes in sports such as football and soccer can tear their posterior cruciate ligament when they fall on a bent knee with their foot pointed down. The shinbone hits the ground first, and it moves backward. Being tackled when your knee is bent also can cause this injury.

PCL injuries can also result from a blow to the knee while it is flexed, or bent. This includes landing hard during sports or a fall, or from a car accident. Any trauma to the knee, whether minor or severe, can cause a knee ligament injury. Also, a direct blow to the front of the knee (such as a bent knee hitting a dashboard in a car crash, or a fall onto a bent knee in sports)

How is PCL Posterior Cruciate Ligament Tears Treated?

Treatment depends on the extent of your injury and whether it just happened or if you've had it for a while. In most cases, surgery isn't required. Once the injury has been correctly diagnosed, 2 modes of treatment may be recommended, conservative treatment or surgery.

Conservative Treatment

If you have injured just your posterior cruciate ligament, your injury may heal quite well without surgery. Your doctor may recommend simple, nonsurgical or conservative treatment. Conservative treatment is everything that does not include surgery. This is indicated in most posterior cruciate ligament injuries and may consist of ice and heat treatment, electrotherapy, e.g., TENS and ultrasound, manual therapy and exercises.

Advice on a specific rehabilitative exercise program which may include quadriceps and hamstring strengthening, gait re-education and balance training using wobble boards. A knee support or brace can be used in the early to mid stages. Hinged knee braces will provide the most support for knee ligament injuries.

RICE: When you are first injured, the RICE method - rest, ice, gentle compression and elevation — can help speed your recovery.

Immobilization: Your doctor may recommend a brace to prevent your knee from moving. To further protect your knee, you may be given crutches to keep you from putting weight on your leg.

Medications: Over-the-counter pain relievers, such as ibuprofen (Advil, Motrin IB, others) or naproxen sodium (Aleve), can help relieve pain and reduce swelling.

Physical therapy: For low-grade injuries to the PCL, Dr. Stone may recommend a regimen of physical therapy. The program will focus initially on immobilizing the PCL and reducing the swelling and inflammation associated with the injury. Specific exercises will be introduced to restore the function of the knee and to strengthen the supporting muscle groups that support the knee.

Surgical Treatment

A lesser proportion of PCL injuries require surgical intervention. However in more severe cases, in particular, those in which other structures within the knee joint have been injured, surgery may be recommended. Surgery may also be indicated if the conservative management has not aided the stability of the knee sufficiently over a period.

Following a thorough examination of all other compartments of the knee for any other damaged tissue, the posterior cruciate ligament (PCL) is well probed to determine the integrity of the remaining fibers. If there is adequate, good quality tissue with some of the remaining fibers still attached, then a PCL repair is performed. If the tissue is irreparably damaged, a reconstruction using a donor graft is performed.

Complete tears of the PCL are best treated with anatomic reconstruction. In the past, isolated PCL injuries were left alone due to the fact that the reconstruction techniques were not reliable. However, patients with torn PCLs develop medial compartment and anterior compartment arthritis, and the knee does not feel stable. With our technique, anatomic PCL reconstruction using sterilized allograft bone patellar tendon bone grafts has led to stable athletic knees.

In general, those who have sustained a PCL injury normally have good recovery rates, with most being able to return to sporting activities at the same level as before the injury. However, full recovery from cruciate ligament damage is highly dependent on the ability to adhere to a strict rehabilitation program.

What Are Some Of The Side Effects Associated With The Treatment Of Posterior Cruciate Ligament (PCL) Tears?

Posterior cruciate ligament (PCL) injuries are less common than anterior cruciate ligament injuries. Consequently, there are fewer reported series of

PCL reconstructions. These PCL reconstructions are technically demanding. There are several complications inherent to the technical aspects of PCL reconstruction. Improper graft placement can lead to limited postoperative knee flexion and extension or even graft failure. Selection of poor graft materials such as the medial gastrocnemius and iliotibial band will result in reconstructions that fail to achieve objective stability.

In many cases, other structures within the knee — including other ligaments or cartilage — also are damaged when you injure your posterior cruciate ligament. Depending on how many of these structures are damaged, you might have some long-term knee pain and instability. You might also be at higher risk of eventually developing arthritis in your affected knee.

In addition to standard risks associated with all orthopedic surgical procedures, posterior cruciate ligament (PCL) reconstruction poses some relatively unique potential complications. These complications arise from a combination of several factors: the relative infrequency of PCL injuries, the lack of knowledge and experience in treating them, the proximity of neurovascular structures to the PCL, and the technically demanding nature of reconstructive procedures.

What is Chondromalacia?

Chondromalacia patella (CMP) is referred to as anterior knee pain due to the physical and biomechanical changes. The articular cartilage of the posterior surface of the patella is going through degenerative changes which manifests as a softening, swelling, fraying, and erosion of the hyaline cartilage underlying the patella and sclerosis of the underlying bone. It is inflammation of the underside of the patella and softening of the cartilage. Chondromalacia patellae is a term sometimes treated synonymously with patellofemoral pain syndrome. Also, chondromalacia patella is weakening and softening of the cartilage on the underside of the kneecap (patella). It is felt that the degeneration of this particular cartilage occurs because of improper alignment of the kneecap in relation to the bone of the thigh, the femur. Knee pain from irritation of this degenerated cartilage during activities is often referred to as patellofemoral syndrome. Chondromalacia patella is one of the most common causes of knee pain, especially in women.

Chondromalacia can affect any joint, but the most common location is inside the knee. It usually begins as a small area of softened cartilage behind the kneecap (patella) that can be painful. Eventually, more of the cartilage softens, and the softened cartilage can crack or shred into a mass of fibers. In severe cases, the damaged cartilage can wear away completely, down to the undersurface of the kneecap. If this happens, the exposed kneecap's bony surface can grind painfully against other knee bones. Also, bits of cartilage can float inside the joint, further irritating the cells that line the joint. In response, these cells produce fluid inside the joint (called a joint effusion).

Patients with chondromalacia patellae usually present with anterior knee pain on walking up or downstairs. Additionally, there may be knee pain when kneeling or squatting or after sitting for long periods of time. Knee stiffness, crepitus, and effusions may also be present. In some cases, a history of patellar dislocation may be present.

The most common symptom of chondromalacia is a dull, aching pain in the front of your knee, behind your kneecap. This pain can get worse when you go up or downstairs. It also can flare up after you have been sitting in one position for a long time. For example, your knee may be painful and stiff when you stand up after watching a movie or after a long trip in a car or plane.

Chondromalacia also can make your knee joint "catch" meaning you suddenly have trouble moving it past a certain point, or "give way" (buckle unexpectedly). These symptoms tend to occur when you bend your knee repeatedly, especially when you go downstairs. In some cases, the painful knee also can appear puffy or swollen. Chondromalacia can cause a creaky sound or grinding sensation when you move your knee. However, creaking sounds during bending do not always mean that cartilage is damaged.

How Common is Chondromalacia in the United States?

Chondromalacia patella is one of the most frequently encountered causes of anterior knee pain among young people. It's the number one cause in the United States with an incidence as high as one in four people. According to Sports Health, 25% of the general population, continues to suffer from runner's knee. When it comes to running, it accounts for up to 40% of knee pain complaints.

Chondromalacia (runner's knee) affects one in four people in the United States. Running is one of the most common causes of chondromalacia, but you should know that it's not the only cause. Any activity that you may be involved in that adds pressure or stress, repeatedly to the joint of your knee can end up causing the condition. This includes cycling, walking, skiing, and even soccer.

Females experienced patellofemoral pain more often than males. The diagnosis of patellofemoral pain increased with age and the 50-59 year-old age group had the most cases.

What Causes Chondromalacia?

Chondromalacia patella often occurs when the undersurface of the kneecap comes in contact with the thigh bone causing swelling and pain. Abnormal knee cap positioning, tightness or weakness of the muscles associated with the knee, too much activity involving the knee, and flat feet may increase the likelihood of chondromalacia patella.

This disease often strikes teenagers and young adults and is believed to be caused by excessive use of the joint, injury, and a forceful blow to the knee.

Females are more prone to acquiring this syndrome. One of the causes is incorrect kneecap position common in a majority of young sufferers. Chondromalacia patella may also signal the onset of kneecap arthritis which usually afflicts people of advanced age. Those at risk of acquiring the disease are those who have a history of dislocations, fractures, or other kneecap injuries.

Many people are surprised to find that their cartilage is damaged because they've never directly injured their knees. However, chondromalacia can be caused by more than an injury or accident. The most common causes include:

- Excessive use of the knees with running, jumping, or any activity that requires heavy use of the knees. Chondromalacia is often called "runner's knee" for this reason. It occurs in people of any age and is common in young, active athletes.

- A kneecap that is out of alignment. If the kneecap isn't in the proper position, the cartilage won't be able to protect it from rubbing. Some people are born with a misalignment of the knee that can cause this issue.

- Weak muscles in the thighs or calves. The leg muscles help support the knee and keep it in place. If they're not strong enough, the knee may slip out of alignment. Even a slight misalignment can gradually wear down the cartilage and cause pain over time.

- A knee injury, such as from an accident, fall or blow to the knee. This could throw the kneecap out of proper alignment or damage the cartilage, or both.

- Another cause is muscles that are not balanced. Strong thigh muscles combined with weaker calf muscles can also push the kneecap out of place.

How is Chondromalacia Treated?

Treatment includes resting the involved knee. Ice and nonsteroidal anti-inflammatory medications (NSAIDs) such as ibuprofen, naproxen, or aspirin may be used to relieve pain following activity that stresses the knee.

Physical therapy to balance the quadriceps and hamstring muscles may be helpful. Taping to realign the kneecap or wearing a brace that has an opening over the kneecap may help control the movement of the kneecap and diminish symptoms. Orthotics (specially fitted shoe inserts) may add support especially for those with flat feet.

If the conservative treatment options mentioned above do not relieve the symptoms or there are signs of arthritis developing, surgery may be an option. This may involve arthroscopic surgery (surgery using a camera inserted through a small opening).

People who have knee pain or symptoms of chondromalacia should see their doctor. Early treatment can prevent further damage to the cartilage and alleviate pain. Typically, noninvasive treatments for chondromalacia are successful. They include:

Avoiding activities that cause pain: Many people must avoid stairs if climbing them causes pain. Instead, they should do exercises that are comfortable. This may help prevent further damage to the cartilage.

Anti-inflammatory medicines: Nonsteroidal anti-inflammatory medications (NSAIDS) are frequently recommended by orthopedics for curing knee pain. This is effective for knee pain that occurs as a result of tendonitis, arthritis, and bursitis.

Physical therapy: There are very effective forms of treatment for the common knee injuries and can be performed in consultation with a physiotherapist. The physical therapy can assist in augmenting strength, reclaiming mobility and facilitating daily return activity with ease.

Cortisone injections: These are normally used to inject cortisone into the knee joint to lessen or reduce inflammation. One should keep in mind that Cortisone is not a knee pain reducing medication; it's only a potent anti-inflammatory medication.

Ice and heat application: Ice packs and heat applications are generally used as a first response to a knee injury. Alternating between hot and cold packs can be of assistance to reduce inflammation and pain in the knee.

Stretching: Basic stretching exercises that focus on muscles and tendons around the knee joint are of great help to reduce the knee pain. Also, walking and swimming are good options to strengthen the legs and keep the muscles strong without stressing the knee.

Medications: Ibuprofen or naproxen are often recommended to help relieve pain and inflammation in the cartilage.

Working toward a healthy weight: Being overweight can be damaging to knee cartilage. Losing weight can relieve stress on the knee joint.

Finally, surgery will only be needed if the pain is severe and other treatments haven't helped. During surgery, the surgeon may remove the rough surface of cartilage to reduce pain. They may also be able to release tight tendons and ligaments. This can help to align the kneecap.

Also, the prognosis of chondromalacia is good, and the condition usually improves with therapy and the use of NSAIDS. If surgery is required, this is often successful.

What Are Some Of The Side Effects Associated With The Treatment of Chondromalacia?

If chondromalacia isn't treated, it can lead to patella-femoral arthritis. This occurs when the cartilage gets severely worn away by damage. Once the cartilage is lost, it cannot grow back. In severe cases, the bones may directly rub together. If this happens, the pain may be debilitating and may be felt while resting.

Risk factors that may increase the risk of developing chondromalacia patella include abnormal positioning of the kneecap; tightness or weakness of the thigh muscles; overuse from activities such as running, jumping or twisting, skiing or playing soccer; flat feet; previous injury or trauma to the kneecap.

Other possible complications include:

- Failure of physical therapy and NSAIDs use to effect pain relief

- Surgical complications include infection, the absence of pain relief, and worsened pain

CHAPTER 19

COSMETICS AND REGENERATIVE MEDICINE

Introduction

Cosmetology is the study and application of beauty treatment. The difference between cosmetic and aesthetic is that cosmetic is imparting or improving the beauty, particularly the beauty of the complexion while aesthetic is concerned with beauty, artistic impact, or appearance. This chapter includes details about cosmetics, the facial features which determine beauty, the impact of aging on facial anatomy, the best practice standards for injection techniques of dermal fillers and the facial as well as skin pathologies that require cosmetic treatments.

1. What are facial feature ideals including the proportions and dimensions that are determined to create beauty?

The perfect face included these key features:

- The length of the face equals the length of three noses.

- Width of an eye in between the eyes.

- Upper and lower lips are the same widths.

- Symmetrical eyebrows conforming to the line of the nose.

- Space from the lower eyelid to the upper eyelid is the same as space between the upper eyelid and eyebrow.

- Eyebrow begins on the same line as the corner of the eye nearest to the nose.

- The width of the face across the cheeks is equal to two lengths of the nose. (Russell)

2. What are the facial changes that occur due to aging in both female and male patients of all cultures?

Despite variation in lifestyle and environment, the first signs of the human facial aging show between the ages of 20–30 years. It is a cumulative process of changes in the skin, soft tissue, and skeleton of the face. Despite individual variation in onset and progression, human facial aging shows a common pattern of morphological, histological, and dermatological changes, as addressed in numerous biomedical studies. Bone tissues along the orbital rim, especially superomedial and inferolateral, have been shown to recede with increasing age, while the central orbital parts remain relatively stable throughout life. This contributes to a more prominent medial fat pad, elevated medial brows, and the typical lengthening of the lid-cheek junction in older age(Mendelson and Wong). Retrusion of the bony midface and the maxilla in adds to building and deepening the nasolabial folds and to increasing facial flatness. The lengthening of the nose results from an enlargement of the piriform aperture as the bony edges recede, especially in the ascending process of the maxilla. Together with reduced soft-tissue laxity, this also leads to a drooping nose tip. Moreover, the height and length of the mandible decrease in older ages, whereas the mandibular angle increases.

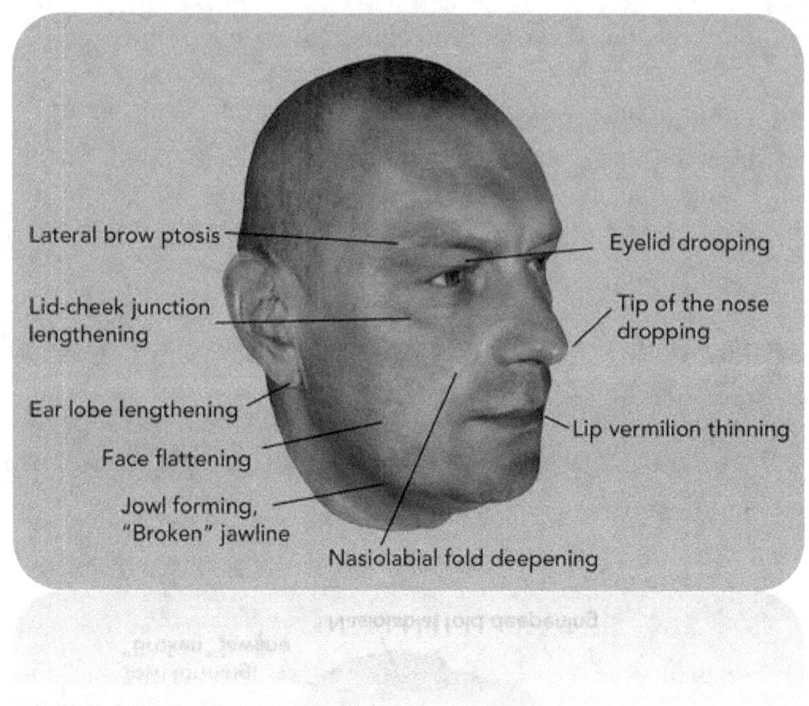

Figure 1

Image link: https://onlinelibrary.wiley.com/cms/attachment/8a4bfbdb-2d47-48a7-98bb-299a54ce50a6/ajpa23878-fig-0001-m.png

Collagen fibers are responsible for the resilience and main mass of the dermis. Males have more collagen than females throughout adult. With increasing age, the amount, quality, and type of collagen change. In both sexes, total skin collagen and skin thickness decrease. Yet, especially after menopause, collagen becomes reduced both in the skin and bone of female faces. Many societies in East and Southeast Asia are among the most rapidly aging societies in the world surpassing many European and American societies. Specifically, aspects of facial contrast decrease with age in Caucasian women, and Caucasian female faces with higher contrast look younger. The main changes in facial skin color with age are related to chronic sun exposure which causes an overall darkening of the skin in all racial skin types; although some minor modifications of the skin color with age have been reported to be specific to one race or another. (Flament et al.)

3. What is the pharmacology of the various Botulinum Toxins available for aesthetic and therapeutic use?

Botulinum toxin, also known as Botox, is produced by Clostridium botulinum, a gram-positive anaerobic bacterium. Botulinum toxin has a well-defined role among dermatologists for the treatment of facial wrinkling, brow position, and palmar and axillary hyperhidrosis. Botulinum toxin blocks the release of acetylcholine from the presynaptic terminal of the neuromuscular junction. (Aoki) Botulinum toxins are, as a group, among the most potent neuromuscular toxins known, yet they are clinically useful in the management of conditions associated with muscular and glandular over-activity. The therapeutic uses of botulinum toxins include spasticity, inappropriate body sphincter contraction, eye movement disorders, hyperkinetic movement disorders, autonomic disturbances, cosmetology and pain syndromes. Botulinum toxin type A (BTA) can be used for facial aesthetics. The 3 currently available BTA types include onabotulinumtoxinA, abobotulinumtoxinA and incobotulinumtoxinA. The clinical use of botulinum toxin to selectively depress skeletal muscle activity in treating facial spasmodic disorders began in the 1970s. Its aesthetic uses were discovered incidentally but have dramatically changed the landscape of facial rejuvenation. In 1989, the FDA approved the use of onabotulinum toxin A (Botox) for the treatment of facial spasmodic disorders. In that same year, Clark and Berris reported the use of Botox as a treatment for facial asymmetry resulting from iatrogenic facial nerve damage during rhytidectomy. (Clark and Berris) This use is widely considered the first aesthetic use of botulinum neurotoxin.

4. What are the "best practice" standards for injection techniques for all of the Botulinum Toxins and their dosing equivalents for the

treatment of facial muscle rebalancing for youthful expression?

The best practice standards for injection techniques for all of the Botulinum Toxins incorporate:

When injecting botulinum toxin, a half-inch 32-gauge needle (Air-Tite Products) minimizes injection discomfort. In the periorbital areas, botulinum is injected in an oblique manner to the skin to lessen the chance of deep injections or even injury should a patient suddenly move. (Strobl et al.)Pinching upward or gently rubbing the adjacent skin during injection minimizes patient discomfort by distracting the patient during the injection and "confusing" the sensory sensation of the injection.

Botox is most commonly used on the wrinkles between the eyebrows. This area is called the glabella. The practice standard for injection technique for the botulinum toxins in glabella is:

Botulinum toxin is supplied as a powder and is reconstituted at the time of treatment into a solution using sterile normal saline. Dilution volumes range from 1 to 4 mL per 100-unit vial. The botulinum toxin dose injected into glabellar complex muscles for the treatment of frown lines is based on the specific botulinum toxin product used and the mass of the target muscles. The targeted glabellar complex muscles can be identified by having the patient actively frown, and injections are placed into the contracted muscles. Small volumes of botulinum toxin solution are injected, typically 1 mL or less, using a 30-gauge, 1-inch needle. There are five injection sites, one injection in the procerus muscle and two in each of the corrugator supercilii muscles. Botulinum toxin is commonly used to treat other lines in the upper one-third of the face, such as horizontal forehead lines with injection in the frontalis muscle, and crow's feet with injection in the lateral orbicularis oculi muscles. Localized burning or stinging sensation during injection is commonly reported and resolves within a few minutes.

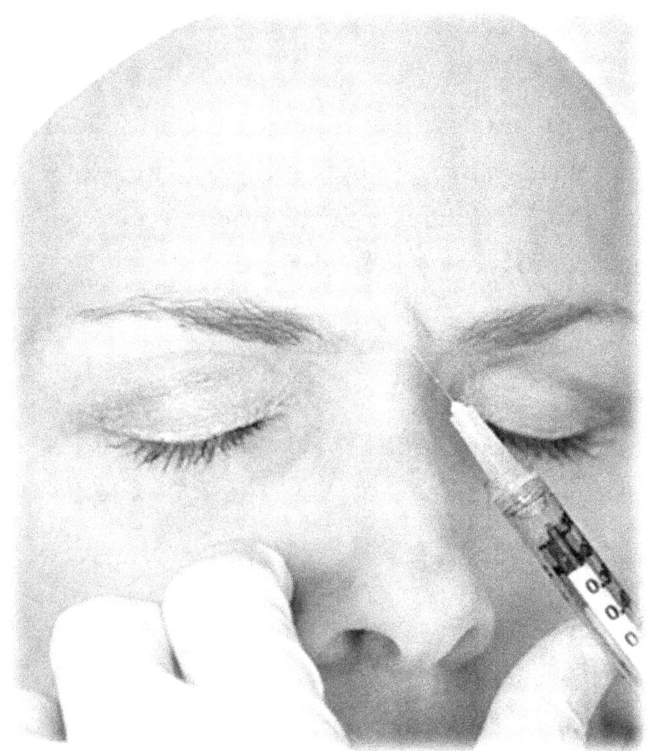

Figure 2

Image link: https://www.aafp.org/afp/2014/0801/afp20140801p168-f6.jpg

5.   What areas are commonly treated? (frown lines, brow furrows, brow elevation, crow's feet, bunny lines, lip lines, nasolabial folds, marionette folds, aging jawline, and aging neck)

☐ **Forehead Lines:** Frontalis Muscle. Injections of 5 to 25u will usually be adequate. Horizontal lines (or "pleats") are injected every 1 1/2 to 2 cm but high enough from the brow to prohibit brow ptosis.

☐   **Glabella/Frown Lines:** Corrugator Supercilii and Procerus muscles. Injections of 20 to 25u will usually be adequate. Approximately 5 injections can be given in this area, between 2 and 2.5u per corrugator and 2.5u into the procerus. The injector should take care not to inject pass the middle of the brow, or above or past the pupil. This could lead to brow ptosis.

☐ **Crow's Feet (Lateral Orbital Lines):** Orbicularis Oculi and Procerus Muscles. Injections of 5 to 15u will usually be adequate. The pleats are injected with 2.5u. The injector should take care to avoid lid ptosis by injecting too close to the eyelids themselves.

☐ **Bunny Lines (Transverse nasal):** Injections of 5 to 25u will usually be adequate.

☐ **Peri-oral Lines (Smoker's Lines):** Orbicularis Oris Muscle. 5u per line will usually be adequate.

☐ **Marionette Lines:** Depressor Anguli Oris and/or Trangularis Muscles

☐ **Mentalis Dysfunction (Chin "Dents"):** Mentalis Muscle (especially after a failed chin augmentation surgery; augmentation mentoplasty). For a standard treatment, 20u of Botox can be injected into various points in the Mentalis to relax the mentalis muscle and prevent visible contour irregularities.

☐ **Vertical Platysma Bands:** Platysma Muscle

6. What are the incidence, prevalence, and pathophysiology of hyperhidrosis?

In Hyperhydrosis or Hyperhidrosis (excessive sweating) BOTOX® can be used to control hyperhidrosis by blocking the release of acetylcholine. Acetylcholine is the body's chemical that stimulates the sweat glands.

- Armpits: Axillary

- Palms: Palmaris

- Soles of the Feet: Plantaris

Hyperhidrosis is thought to affect 2.8% of the US population and can be of primary or secondary origin. (Strutton et al.) Primary hyperhidrosis is usually bilateral, symmetric, and focal. The most common focal sites include, but are not limited to, the palms, soles, and axillae. Secondary hyperhidrosis is usually caused by an underlying medical condition or medication. Secondary hyperhidrosis must be ruled out before a diagnosis of primary hyperhidrosis is made.

Prevalence and incidence of hyperhidrosis

Current results estimate the prevalence of hyperhidrosis at 4.8 %, which represents approximately 15.3 million people in the United States. (Augustin et al.) The prevalence rate is highest among 18–39 years old (8.8 %) and lowest among adults 65+ years old and children/adolescents. (Moraites, Vaughn and Hill) Of these, 70 % report severe excessive sweating in at least one body area. In spite of this, only 51 % have discussed their excessive sweating with a healthcare professional. Prevalence estimates that include both primary and secondary hyperhidrosis range from 13.9 % in Japan, 16.3 % in Germany, 16.7 % in Vancouver, 18.4 % in Shanghai, and 20.3 % in Sweden. (Fujimoto, Kawahara and Yokozeki)

Pathophysiology of Hyperhydrosis

Sweat glands in patients with hyperhidrosis are not histopathologically different from those in normal patients, nor is there an increase in the number or size of glands. The condition is caused by hyperfunction of the sweat glands rather than hypertrophy. Patients with primary hyperhidrosis have a higher-than-normal basal level of sweat production as well as an increased response to normal stimuli such as emotional or physical stress. (Schick)

7. What are various facial fillers available for aesthetic enhancement including autologous fat, cell augmented fat, the various collagens

(Zyderm, Zyplast, Cosmoderm, Cosmoplast, Evolence), the various hyaluronans (Restylane, Perlane, Juvederm, Prevelle, Hydrelle), poly-L-Lactic acid (Sculptra), calcium hydroxyl appetite (Radiesse), and silicone and stem cell therapy?

The facial fillers available for aesthetic enhancement include:

Autologous Fat

The autologous fat transfer (AFT) or lipofilling is used as a potentially superior facial filler with numerous studies reporting on the promising results besides minimal side effects. The autologous fat possesses facial rejuvenating properties ie, volume enhancement, improving skin trophicity, decreasing wrinkles.

Collagens

Type 1 collagen loss in the dermis is one of the primary causes of wrinkles seen in aged skin. Dermal fillers using type 1 collagen derived from bioengineered skin are now being used to treat facial wrinkles. These fillers, known by the trade names of **CosmoDerm** and **CosmoPlast**, can be used alone or in combination with hyaluronic acid fillers. (Bauman) The cosmoderm and cosmoplast and are harvested from bioengineered human skin. The benefit of collagen-based dermal fillers is decreased downtime, decreased bruising, decreased pain on injection, and the ability to return lost structural components to aged skin. Many aesthetic physicians are beginning to use collagen- and hyaluronic-containing fillers in combination to replace both of these natural components of the skin that are lost during the aging process. **Zyderm I** was approved by the FDA in 1981. (Tromovitch, Stegman and Glogau)It was followed by two additional formulations of bovine collagen Zyderm II and Zyplast. Zyderm I is injected superficially in the upper dermis whereas zyderm II and Zyplast are injected in the mid-dermal plane. They have limited cosmetic satisfaction.

Hyaluronans

Juvéderm and *Restylane* are two types of *dermal fillers* used for the treatment of wrinkles. Both injections use a gel made with hyaluronic acid to plump up the *skin*. (Allemann and Baumann) These are noninvasive procedures. No surgery is required. The first HA filler in the United States was Restylane. Restylane received its FDA approval in the United States in December 2003. Restylane's FDA approval is for mid-to-deep dermal implantation for the correction of moderate-to-severe facial wrinkles and folds, such as nasolabial folds. The second product released in the United States, which was in the Restylane family, is known as Perlane.

Juvederm is a cosmetic treatment referred to as a filler. It's used to restore facial contours and improve signs of aging. It's an injectable dermal filler with a base of hyaluronic acid. It's a treatment that focuses on the face, specifically the cheeks, lips, and around the mouth. The procedure to inject the product takes 15 to 60 minutes. It's one of the most common nonsurgical cosmetic procedures done in the U.S

Hydrelle is a cross-linked hyaluronic acid-based dermal, facial filler, in injectable gel form. Cross-linking is a process used to make hyaluronic acid into a gel product, which can be injected into the dermis, for a longer-lasting effect on the skin. (Smith and Cockerham)

Prevelle

Silk is an injectable dermal filler used to treat moderate to severe wrinkles and facial folds. (Kablik et al.) This is one of the newer injectable soft tissue fillers that was approved by the FDA in March 2008.

poly-L-Lactic acid (Sculptra),

Sculptra Aesthetic is a poly-L-lactic acid (PLLA)–based treatment that works deep within the skin to help stimulate collagen production. Unlike hyaluronic acid fillers, Sculptra Aesthetic helps stimulates the skin's own natural collagen production. (Lacombe)

Radiesse

(Bioform Inc, USA) is a sterile, latex-free, non-pyrogenic, semi-solid, cohesive subdermal, injectable facial implant, whose principal component is synthetic calcium hydroxylapatite, a biocompatible material with over 20 years of use in medicine. Radiesse has FDA approval for esthetic facial augmentation in the US. Such approval includes the long-lasting correction of moderate to severe facial wrinkles and folds and the treatment of facial fat loss due to immunodeficiency virus infection. (Jacovella et al.)

Silicone

The advantage of medical-grade silicone as a filler is that it is permanent. When used to smooth lines and remove wrinkles it will not have to be done again. That said, there is a reason it has not been approved for this use by the Food and Drug Administration. Many doctors think as a dermal filler, silicone is unpredictable, its removal after use is difficult, and that the risk of complications is too serious. Those complications can include minor problems like bruising, swelling, and pain, or major problems like skin necrosis, infection, allergic reaction, or the formation of hard nodules. (Buck II, Alam and Kim)

Stem cell filler

The use of stem cells in the cosmetic industry for facial rejuvenation is a relatively recent development. Stem cell filler is injected into the face just like any standard filler. The difference is that 15 to 20 ml or more of stem cell material can be prepared and injected into the face in just one 30 minute session. The stem cells can be injected at various levels within the facial tissues, ranging from very superficial lines of the upper lips and crows feet to deeper nasolabial folds and marionette lines as well as hollow cheeks and temples. Patients often notice a healthy, youthful glow to their facial skin immediately following treatment. (Moseley, Zhu and Hedrick)

8. What are basic dermatology and the dermatologic conditions requiring aesthetic enhancement including lentigines (brown spots), telangiectasias (red spots), wrinkles, elastosis (skin laxity), melasma, cellulite, acne, dysplasia, unwanted hair and unwanted veins?

Lentigines (brown spots)

As an individual gets older, they might notice brown or black spots appear on their skin. These spots are especially common on sun-exposed areas like the face and the backs of hands. They're called lentigines, or liver spots. It's called lentigo because the spots can resemble lentils in color. A lentigo can grow very slowly over many years, or it can appear suddenly. Multiple spots are called lentigines. Treatment is given to lighten or remove lentigines for aesthetic reasons. Following are the number of treatments for lentigines:

- medicines such as bleaching creams containing hydroquinone or retinoids (tretinoin)

- chemical peels

- laser or intense pulse light therapy to destroy melanocytes

- freezing (cryotherapy) to destroy melanocytes (Ortonne et al.)

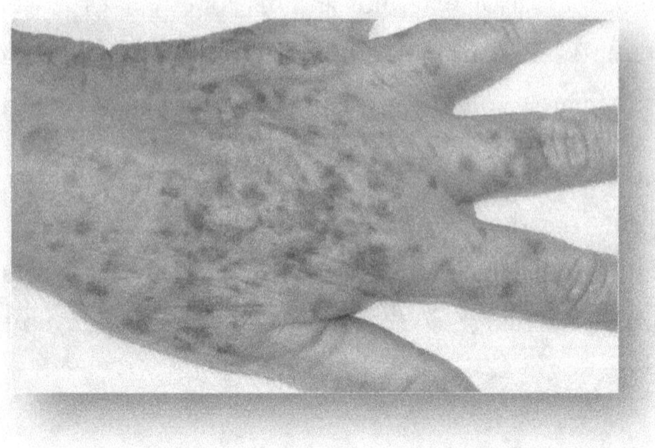

Figure 3

Image link: http://complexi-light.com/wp-content/uploads/2016/01/age-spots-1.jpg

Telangiectasias (red spots)

Telangiectasia is a condition in which widened venules (tiny blood vessels) cause threadlike red lines or patterns on the skin. These patterns, or telangiectases, form gradually and often in clusters. They're sometimes known as "spider veins" because of their fine and weblike appearance. They are common in areas that are easily seen (such as the lips, nose, eyes, fingers, and cheeks). (Guttmacher, Marchuk and White Jr)Treatment:

- <u>laser therapy</u>: laser targets the widened vessel and seals it (this usually involves little pain and has a short recovery period)

- surgery: widened vessels can be removed (this can be very painful and may lead to a long recovery)

- <u>sclerotherapy</u>: focuses on causing damage to the inner lining of the blood vessel by injecting it with a chemical solution that causes a blood clot that collapses, thickens, or scars the venule (there's usually no recovery needed, although there may be some

temporary exercise restrictions)

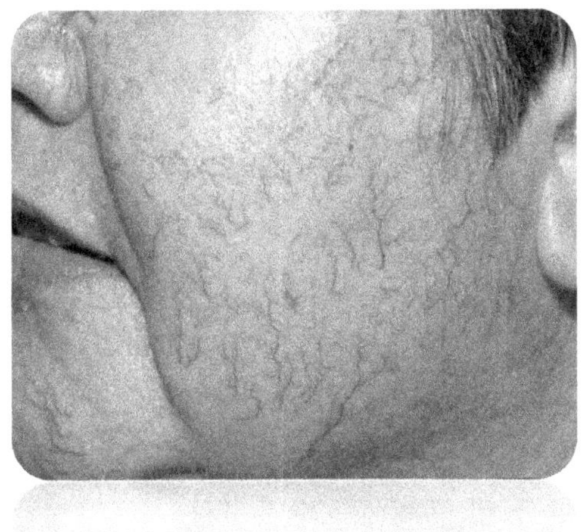

Fig A, link: https://lianhealth.om/wp-content/uploads/2019/07/TelangiectasiaFace.jpg

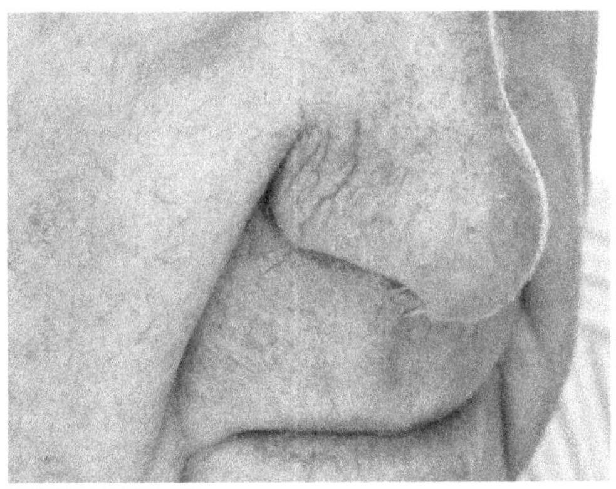

Figure 4, 5 (A, B)

Fig B, link: https://2rdnmg1qbg403gumla1v9i2h-wpengine.netdna-ssl.com/wp-content/uploads/sites/3/2017/09/SpiderVeins-650x450.jpg

Wrinkles

Wrinkles are creases, folds, or ridges in the skin. They normally appear as people get older, but they can also develop after spending a long time in the water. The first wrinkles to appear on a person's face tend to occur as a result of facial expressions. Sun damage, smoking, dehydration, some medications, and environmental and genetic factors affect when and where people will develop wrinkles. Treatment:

The two main types of wrinkles are surface lines and deep furrows.

Most basic wrinkle treatments, if they have any effect, tend to help reduce the fine lines. For deeper creases, there are more aggressive techniques, such as plastic surgery or injections of fillers.

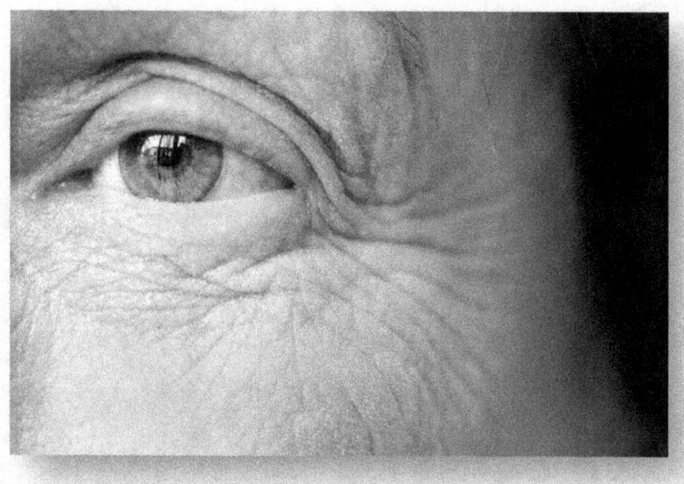

Figure 6

Image link:

https://img.webmd.com/dtmcms/live/webmd/consumer_assets/site_images/articles/health_tools/visual_guide_wrinkles_slideshow/1800ss_getty_rf_crows_feet.jpg?resize=650px:*

Elastosis (Skin laxity)

Loss of skin elasticity is known as elastosis. Elastosis causes skin to look saggy, crinkled, or leathery. Areas of the skin exposed to the sun can get solar elastosis. These parts of the body may look more weathered than those protected from sun exposure. Treatment:

Numerous treatment options are available for photoaged skin, including dermabrasion, topical application of retinoic acid, carbon dioxide laser resurfacing, hyaluronic acid injection into the dermis, imiquimod, tacrolimus ointment, and topical estrogen therapy.

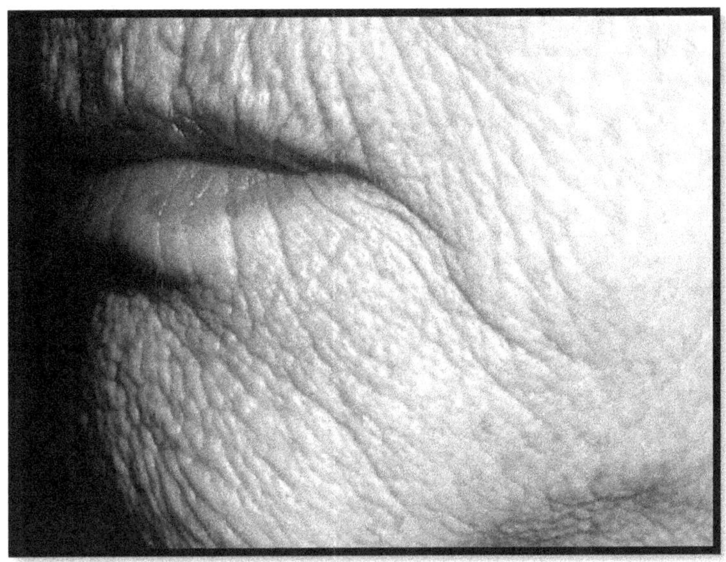

Figure 7

Image link: https://medicalpoint.org/wp-content/uploads/2014/12/solar-elastosis-pictures.jpg

Melasma

Melasma is a common pigmentation disorder that causes brown or gray patches to appear on the skin, primarily on the face. The most common areas for melasma to appear on the face include the bridge of the nose, the forehead, the cheeks, the upper lip. Treatment for melasma includes hydroquinone, tretinoin and corticosteroids.

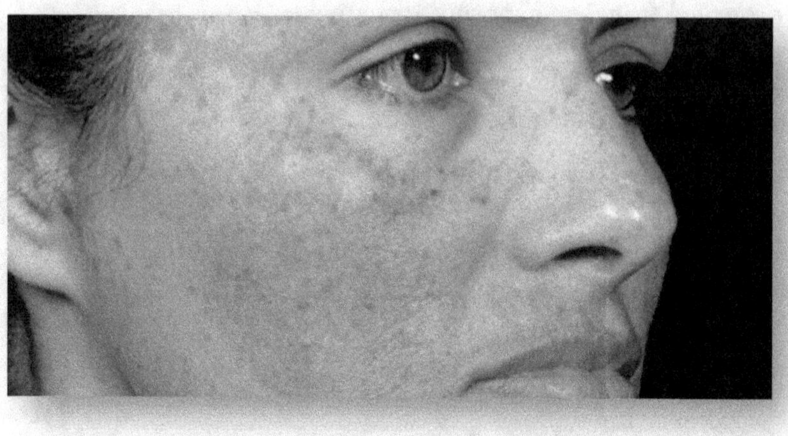

Figure 8

Image link: https://drpimplepopper.com/wp-content/uploads/2017/09/melasma-1100x858-1100x550.jpg

Cellulite

Cellulite is a term for the formation of lumps and dimples in the skin. Common names for cellulite are orange-peel skin, cottage-cheese skin, hail damage, and the mattress phenomenon. Cellulite can affect both men and women, but it is more common in females, due to the different distributions of fat, muscle, and connective tissue. Treatment includes Acoustic wave therapy, Laser treatment, Subcision, Vacuum-assisted precise tissue release Carboxytherapy Endermologie, Ionithermie cellulite reduction treatment, Radiotherapy, Laser-assisted liposuction, Ultrasonic liposculpting, retinol and caffeine.

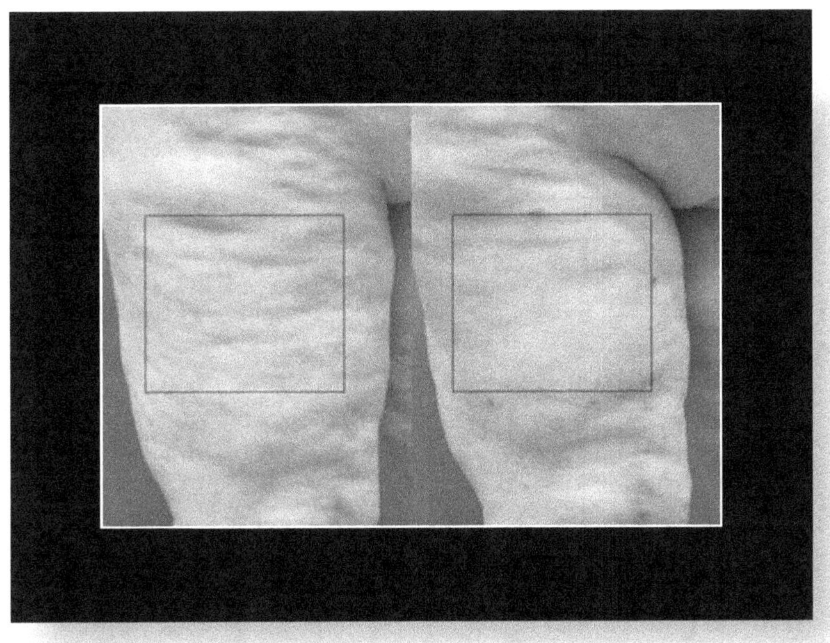

Figure 9

Image link: https://www.builtlean.com/wp-content/uploads/2013/07/cellulite-treatment.jpg

Acne

Acne, also known as acne vulgaris, is a long-term skin disease that occurs when hair follicles are clogged with dead skin cells and oil from the skin. It is characterized by blackheads or whiteheads, pimples, oily skin, and possible scarring. Treatment includes **Resorcinol, Benzoyl peroxide, Salicylic acid, Sulfur, Retin-A: Azelaic acid.**

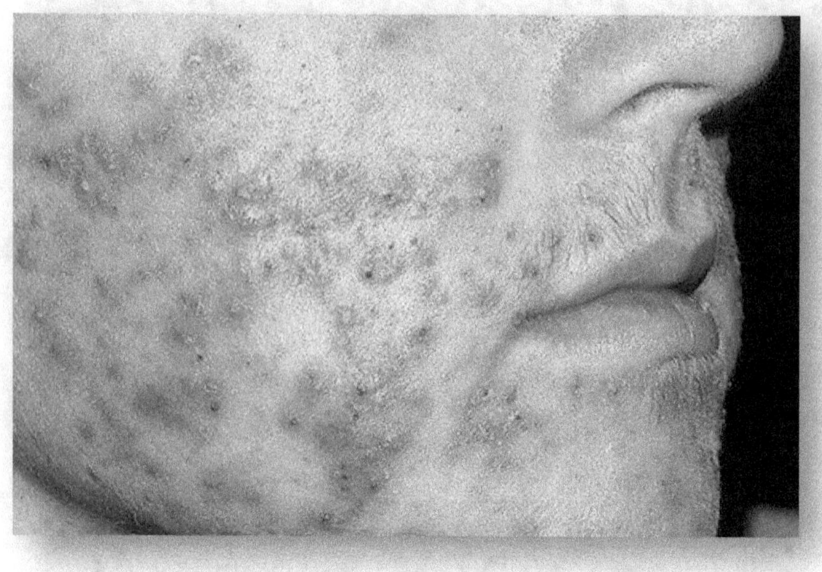

Figure 10

Image link: https://images.medicinenet.com/images/slideshow/boils_s4_cystic_acne.jpg

Dysplasia

Median facial dysplasia (MFD) is a distinct and unique disorder of the craniofacial region that is characteristic of deficient midfacial structures with the addition of a unilateral or bilateral cleft lip with or without a cleft palate. Treatment: surgery.

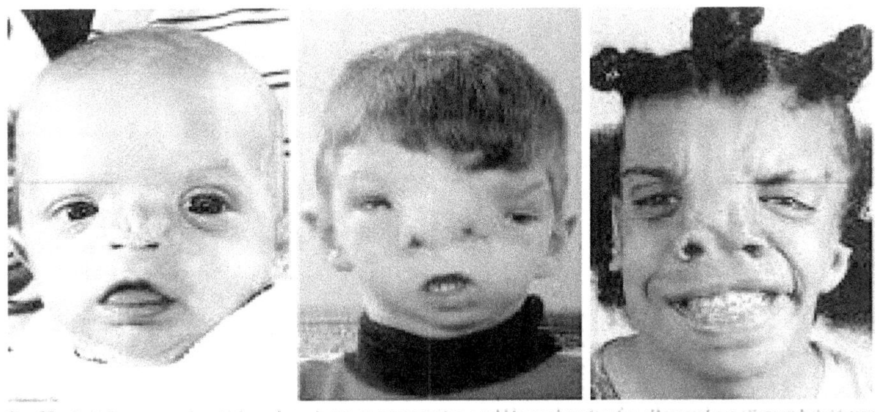

Figure 11

Image link:
https://d3i71xaburhd42.cloudfront.net/2347fd766f06862436d7bfb09a34f7dd2f0139f7/7-
Figure12-1.png

Unwanted hair

All women produce some testosterone, but higher than normal levels may increase your sex drive, affect your menstrual cycle and produce excess **facial** and **body hair.** excess facial hair may be caused by medicines, such as minoxidil which is taken for high blood pressure, congenital adrenal hyperplasia, Cushing's Syndrome, Acromegaly, being overweight or obese, an ovarian tumor and Polycystic ovarian syndrome (PCOs). Treatments: shaving, waxing, bleaching hair removal creams such as Vaniqa, electrolysis and laser hair removal.

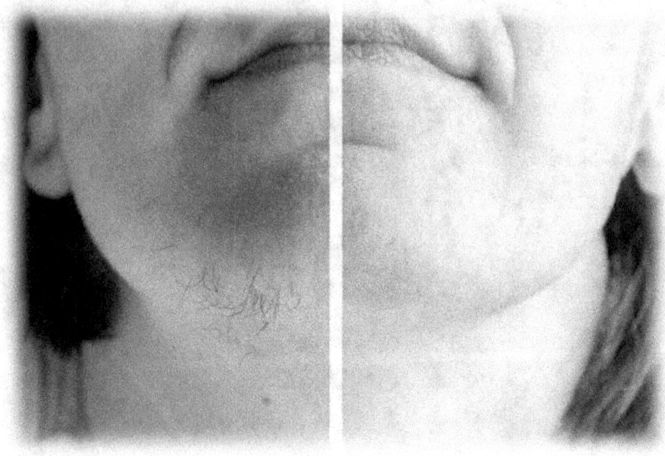

Figure 12

Image link: https://1.bp.blogspot.com/-VfgfN4_mHgM/Xeo4yPg-
4dI/AAAAAAAAKxM/1qrMcHTMl_YT0U98EZSHLn4nVX_F-
9BuACNcBGAsYHQ/s640/0%252BrAQ47g4eOZITZfxVyKG%252BOSnqAC%252BRj2mXh
lbnjp57eYBHX3ZKDh9b2kkhJbHZGtVX0JpXS%252BhENZ8Fd3m04bz%252BZjHdbphMH
DORfiMKdzIfbxr9XciinGOYfefFntqgIzE3u1OY4OQJR_VLobsU0txXHz9vAlt_IkTAfgxOZag
lnQ0groVJ6m%252B4YFtUOC_JO9B1JSs%252BZ3JGCIACH.jpg

Unwanted veins.

One of the main causes of spider **veins** on a patient's **face** is simply the
aging process. Treatment: laser.

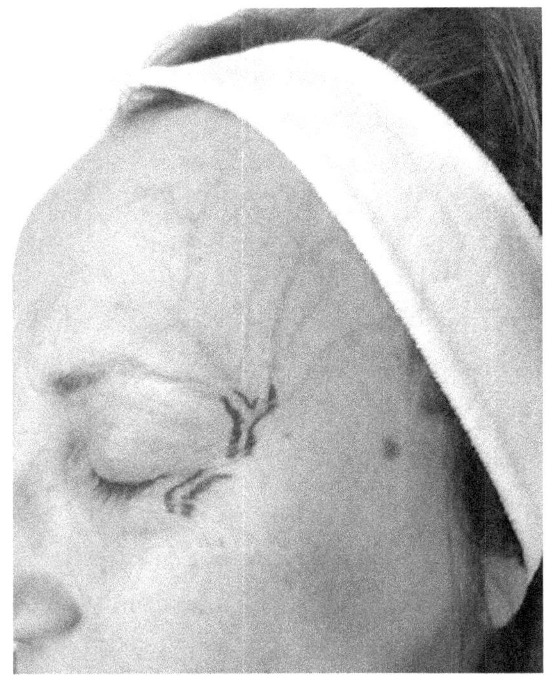

Figure 13

Image link: https://www.thepmfajournal.com/media/14216/pmfadj19-facial-veins_fig-5.png?width=700&height=856

9. What are the laser physics and the principles of laser and light tissue interactions? (This includes photothermolysis, ablative skin resurfacing, non-ablative skin resurfacing, fractional skin resurfacing, photodynamic therapy and photomodulation)

Laser physics

Laser radiation is electromagnetic radiation. The spectrum of electromagnetic radiation ranges from radio wave radiation (long wavelength) via microwave, infrared, visible, and ultraviolet radiation of short-wavelength X-ray and gamma radiation. Laser radiation used in medicine ranges from the UV to the far IR (193-10 600 nm). Wavelength is usually expressed in nanometers (1 nm = 10-9 m). This implies that the visible part of the spectrum of electromagnetic radiation is only a part of the spectrum covered by laser radiation.

Photothermolysis

For many years following the initial studies of the effects of lasers on the skin, the use of lasers was limited to nonselective coagulation and vaporization of tissue. A revolution in the clinical utility of lasers occurred in the early 1980s with the development of the theory of selective photothermolysis. This theory describes the parameters by which light can be used to selectively destroy targets in the skin through the selective absorption of light and spatial confinement of the effect. It matches the specific wavelength of light and heats the tissue and destroys it with a laser without affecting or damaging surrounding tissue.

Ablative skin resurfacing

Ablative laser skin resurfacing is one of the most effective cosmetic procedures for improving aging skin. The procedure works by delivering an intense wavelength of light to the skin, which removes the outer layers of aged or sun-damaged skin.

Non-ablative skin resurfacing

Non-ablative skin rejuvenation uses a laser to improve the appearance of wrinkles, brown spots, and minor scars by creating heat in the skin without injuring the surface of the skin. The heat generated by the laser promotes collagen production which causes the skin to tighten and look young and healthy.

Fractional skin resurfacing

In fractional laser skin resurfacing, a device called a fractional laser delivers precise microbeams of laser light into the lower layers of skin, creating deep, narrow columns of tissue coagulation. Coagulated tissue in the treatment area stimulates a natural healing process that results in the fast growth of healthy new tissue. The procedure can be used on the face, neck, chest, arms and hands.

Photodynamic therapy

Photodynamic therapy (PDT) is a noninvasive technique used in the treatment of various skin disorders. It has been used for skin cancer, precancerous changes of the skin, and for cosmetic purposes in skin rejuvenation.

Photomodulation

Photomodulation using Light-Emitting Diodes (LEDs) is a non-invasive phototherapy technique. It involves using lights with specific wavelengths at a low intensity to stimulate natural biological repair mechanisms. LED photomodulation is a completely natural rejuvenation method that helps to prevent and reverse the signs of aging.

1. What are the potential adverse events when using lasers and light and how to avoid and treat these complications?

Potential adverse events include:

1. Burns,

2. Scarring,

3. Dyspigmentation,

4. Ocular injury, and

5. Infection.

These complications are expected side effects based on the theory of selective photothermolysis and, in some cases, can even be used to the surgeon's advantage, such as when reducing pigmentation in melasma.

Treatment of the complications:

Laser surgeons must be aware of all potential adverse effects associated with cutaneous laser resurfacing so that when one does occur, appropriate interventions can be promptly initiated to prevent further cutaneous damage. Burns are caused by laser and the fastest way to soothe the burning sensation is by cooling the skin down as quickly as possible. After the event of burn a layer of clean cling film is to layover and cover the burn area, however, the cling film must not be wrapped around the burn. Dr. Scales primarily uses oral or IV steroids for severe or acute laser injuries, particularly YAG injuries. For ocular injuries, nonsteroidal anti-inflammatory drugs are used.

> 10. What the licensure requirements and the central role of an aesthetician in an aesthetic practice?

Licensure requirements of an esthetician

To serve in the profession, aestheticians must be licensed in aesthetics by a state cosmetology board. Common licensure requirements include graduation from an approved school and passage of written and practical exams. Some cosmetology boards allow aestheticians to substitute formal education with apprenticeship training to meet the licensure requirements. Maryland, for example, requires candidates to have 600 hours of formal education or 12 months of apprenticeship training. (Warfield)

The central role of aesthetician

Estheticians provide quality skincare services following the best standard practices in the salon, spa, retail, or medical settings. Their job is to enhance the quality of skin through services such as facials, color analysis, microdermabrasion, chemical peels, hair removal, etc.

11. What the potential adverse events with the aesthetic use of chemical peeling agents and how to avoid and manage these complications

Adverse events of chemical peeling agents

The risks, side effects, and complications of chemical peels include scarring, infection, reactivation of herpes simplex infections, and a substantial contrast in the coloration of the treated skin. All patients will have a recuperation period, the length of which depends upon the depth of the peel. (Roberts)

Treatment of complications

The first step in preventing complications is to identify the patients at risk, so that complication can be anticipated, prevented, and if they still happen, treated at the earliest. These patients include those with darker skin type with a tendency to develop post-inflammatory hyperpigmentation; with sensitive skin or history of atopic dermatitis; with dry skin and a reddish hue, with outdoor occupations; with history of photosensitivity or post-inflammatory hyperpigmentation; and on photosensitizing drugs. The pre-peeling precautions include adequate priming of the skin for at least 2-4 weeks prior to peel and discontinuing 3-5 days before the procedure is of vital importance. Priming is done by the application of depigmenting agents such as hydroquinone or retinoic acid and the use of sunscreens. Post-peel precautions include that sun exposure should be avoided and broad-spectrum sunscreen should be used meticulously, calamine lotion in a moisturizing base can be used for stinging sensation. Thorough knowledge about chemical peeling and the risks involved, adequate patient counseling and education, and performing peels with all basic precautions minimize the complications of chemical peels.

12. What is sclerotherapy and its potential uses and adverse risk factors?

Sclerotherapy

Sclerotherapy is a medical procedure used to eliminate varicose veins and spider veins. Sclerotherapy involves an injection of a solution (generally a salt solution) directly into the vein. The solution irritates the lining of the blood vessel, causing it to collapse and stick together and the blood to clot. (Berenguer et al.)

People with spider veins should consider sclerotherapy when:

- the veins are painful

- the legs are sore or feel heavy

- the skin on the legs or feet is patchy or dry

- there is a rash near the veins

The most common negative reactions to sclerotherapy include bruising, redness, and pain near the injected vein.

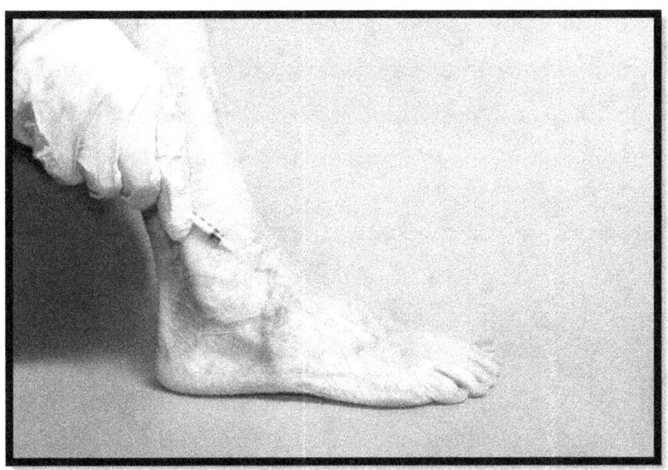

Figure 14

Image link: https://i0.wp.com/cdn-
prod.medicalnewstoday.com/content/images/articles/320/320282/sclerotherapy-being-
performed-on-varicose-veins-in-foot.jpg?w=1155&h=1541

13. What are the toxic ingredients contained in many over the counter products

Dermal filler procedures can be expensive, which has prompted some consumers to turn to the online black market to purchase do-it-yourself fillers. In the last month, there have been multiple reports in media outlets and in the medical literature of dangerous complications resulting from self-injection of fillers by non-health professionals. One risk is that fillers purchased online can contain a variety of nonsterile substances, such as hair gel. When injected, these substances can cause allergic reactions, infections, and the death of skin cells.

14. What are the ingredients in cosmeceutical products including the various retinol, growth factors, peptides, antioxidants, lightening agents, metals, botanicals, vitamins, SPF agents, and their mechanism of action in promoting skin health

Ingredients in cosmeceutical products

Retinols are made from vitamin A, retinol is added to creams that go on the skin. It boosts the amount of collagen the body makes and plumps out skin, reducing fine lines and wrinkles. It also improves skin tone and color and reduces mottled patches.

Growth factors are natural substances made by the skin cells that support the repair of damaged skin, as a result of aging or environmental factors. They promote the formation of collagen and elastin to provide firmness and elasticity.

Peptides are made of amino acids. Peptides are added to skin cosmetics because they can stimulate skin fibroblasts to produce more collagen, elastin, and other proteins in the matrix of the dermis. Boosting these structure proteins makes skin look firmer and fuller.

Antioxidants are naturally occurring vitamins and minerals—like vitamins A, C, E, and green tea—that protect your skin against free radicals.

Lightening agents and skin lighteners use drugs such as steroids and retinoic acid, which comes from vitamin A, as active ingredients. And some skin lighteners use natural ingredients such as kojic acid, a compound that comes from a fungus and arbutin, a compound found in various plants.

Botanicals are powerful plant extracts and oils derived from flowers, herbs, nuts, seeds, roots, and berries. And when harnessed in the right way, they can do wonders for our skin.

Vitamins: Vitamin D is one of the best vitamins for the skin, along with vitamins C, E, and K. The vitamins help make skin looking healthy and youthful.

Spf agents: Sunblock typically refers to opaque sunscreen that is effective at blocking both UVA and UVB rays and uses a heavy carrier oil to resist being washed off. Titanium dioxide and zinc oxide are two minerals that are used in sunblock.

15. What is the appropriate prescription of daily skincare products to promote optimal skin health in your patients and to ensure excellent results with your aesthetic procedures

As the skin grows older, its inherent antiaging mechanisms diminish: defenses weaken, critical processes slow, and the rate of breakdown of key constituents increases. Although cosmetic procedures have a significant positive impact on specific aspects of aging, such as deep wrinkling, sagging, and volume loss, they do not necessarily address the overall quality of the skin. Recommending an at-home skincare regimen based on the patient's individual needs is synergistic with the services cosmetic dermatologists and surgeons provide. Clinically proven products, formulated with the right ingredients for a specific skin concern and delivered in an esthetically appealing system, will both maximize the outcome and increase the longevity of benefits from the treatments provided while empowering the patient to personalize and control their skincare journey.

CHAPTER 20

AESTHETICS AND REGENERATIVE THERAPY

Introduction

Aesthetic dermatology is the treatment for the skin, hair or body that is meant to enhance the appearance of a patient. It is dermatology that is focused on enhancing looks instead of eradicating the disease. In this chapter incidence, prevalence, and morbidity associated with chronic venous insufficiency, risk factors of venous disease, diagnostic tools used for the evaluation of venous insufficiency, role of compression therapy in the treatment of venous disease incidence, prevalence, morbidity, and co-morbidity of obesity worldwide, cellulite and its pathophysiology, and energy-based devices used to treat obesity, localized adiposity, cellulite, and skin laxity have been discussed in detail.

1. **What are the incidence, prevalence, and morbidity associated with chronic venous insufficiency**

Chronic Venous Insufficiency

Chronic venous insufficiency (CVI) is a condition that occurs when the venous wall and/or valves in the leg veins are not working effectively, making it difficult for blood to return to the heart from the legs. CVI causes blood to "pool" or collects in these veins, and this pooling is called stasis. (Eberhardt and Raffetto)

Incidence

Incidence of CVI The annual incidence is 2–6% in women and 1.9% in men. In younger men, the incidence of chronic venous insufficiency is lower than 10%, compared with 30% in similarly aged women. In men older than 50 years, the incidence is 20%, compared with 50% in similarly aged women. Peak incidence occurs in women aged 40-49 years and in men aged 70-79 years. (Modrall et al.)

Prevalence

The prevalence of CVI ranges between 25–40% and 10–20% in women and men, respectively. According to the 2018 survey, the mean incidence of hospital admission for CVI is 92 per 100,000 admissions in the United States. The frequency of venous insufficiency is believed to be higher in Westernized and industrialized nations than in developing nations, most likely because of differences in lifestyle and activity. The prevalence of venous insufficiency increases with age. (Fowkes, Evans and Lee)

Morbidity

More than 30 million people in the United States have some form of chronic venous disease (CVD). The prevalence of CVD is 10 times that of peripheral arterial disease. (Gloviczki et al.)Chronic venous disease is a major source of morbidity (incidence, 92 cases per 100,000 hospital admissions annually. (Heller)

2. **What are the risk factors of venous disease including**

heredity, hormonal influences, lifestyle, and congenital abnormalities?

Risk factors of venous disease:

1. Heredity

2. Hormonal influences

3. Lifestyle

4. Congenital abnormalities

Heredity: There is a strong body of circumstantial evidence that implicates genetics in the etiology and pathology of varicose veins and venous ulcer disease. This suggests inborn genetic traits play a key role in the development of abnormal veins. Moreover, it is also likely that genetic variation, persistent ambulatory venous hypertension and chronic inflammation influence the development of the chronic venous disease. (Krysa, Jones and Van Rij)

Hormonal influences:

In chronic venous insufficiency of the lower limbs sex hormones directly influence disease development through intracellular receptors. The relationship between sex hormones and venous pathology primarily focuses on the increased thrombogenic risk they produce. Female sex hormones may play a predominant role in varicose physiopathology, especially considering the influence of gender and pregnancy on varicose vein development. (Cordts and Gawley)

Lifestyle: A sedentary lifestyle minimizes the pump action of calf muscles on venous return, causing higher venous pressure. CVI occurs more frequently in women who are obese. (Lee et al.)

Congenital abnormalities: Venous insufficiency syndromes are most commonly caused by valvular incompetence in the low-pressure superficial venous system but may also be caused by valvular incompetence in the high-pressure deep venous system (or, rarely, both). In addition, they may result from the congenital absence of venous valves. (Kistner, Eklof and Masuda)

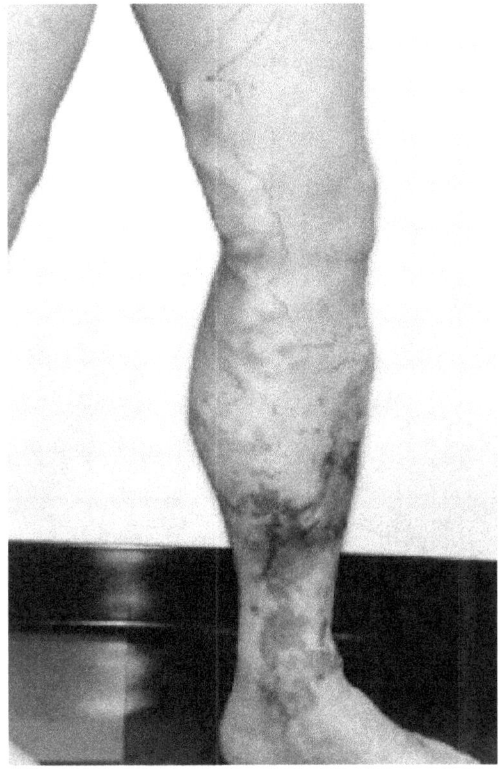

Figure 1

Image link: https://img.medscapestatic.com/pi/meds/ckb/43/28443tn.jpg

3. **What diagnostic tools are used for the evaluation of venous insufficiency including transillumination (veinlite), photoplethysmography (PPG), continuous wave Doppler, and duplex ultrasound?**

The diagnostic tools used for the evaluation of venous

insufficiency include the following:

Transillumination (veinlite):

Veinlite®'s transillumination technology is based on the use of bright, colored LEDs that are positioned directly on the skin's surface during a vein access procedure. As this light passes through the skin, deoxygenated blood absorbs some of the light. The result is a true representation of not only the location of the vein but also the size and depth of the vein. In addition to locating veins, Veinlite also secures them to prevent rolling, aiding technicians in successful vein access. Veinlite is effective in finding veins up to 6mm deep. All Veinlite® device is small and portable to allow for quick access and usage. The simple handheld form factor requires just one technician and no formal training to use. Depending on the model, Veinlite® units cost anywhere between $270-$440. Veinlite® is clinically proven to provide a significant improvement in first-time success rate over any other method. This results in patient satisfaction, technician confidence, and savings in supplies used. The world's only genuine and patented Veinlite® transillumination devices are manufactured in the USA by TransLite LLC. (Katsogridakis et al.)

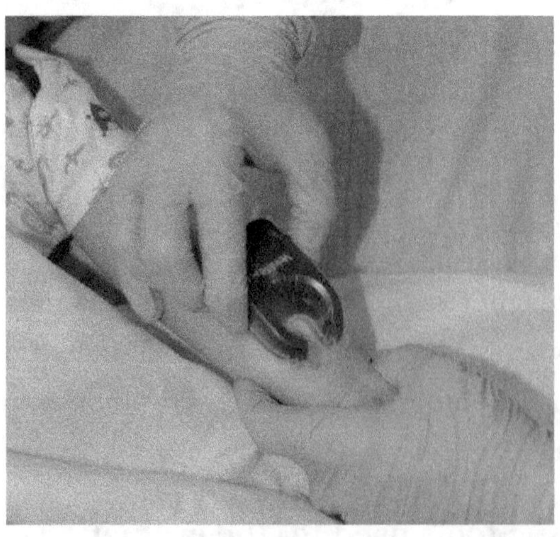

Figure 2: Transilluminator

Image link: https://img.medicalexpo.com/images_me/photo-g/84267-4383679.jpg

Photoplethysmography (PPG):

A photoplethysmogram (PPG) is an optically obtained plethysmogram that can be used to detect blood volume changes in the microvascular bed of tissue. A photoplethysmography (PPG) is often obtained by using a pulse oximeter which illuminates the skin and measures changes in light absorption. PPG detects the change of blood volume by the photoelectric technique, whether transmissive or reflective, to record the volume of blood in the sensor coverage area to form a PPG signal. Indeed, the sensor coverage area includes both veins and arteries, and numerous capillaries. Thus, the PPG signal is a complex mixture of the blood flow in veins and arteries of the cardiovascular circulatory system. A raw PPG signal generally includes pulsatile and non-pulsatile blood volume. (Allen)

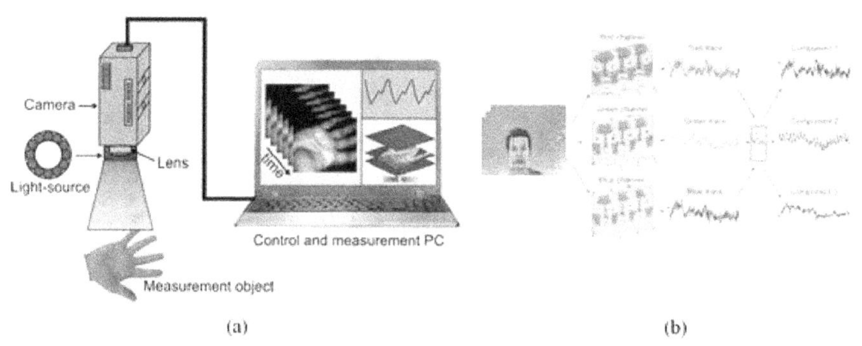

Figure 3: Photoplethysmography

Image link: https://media.springernature.com/lw785/springer-static/image/chp%3A10.1007%2F978-3-319-69362-0_6/MediaObjects/421117_1_En_6_Fig3_HTML.gif

Continuous wave Doppler:

Continuous-wave Doppler utilizes continuous transmission and reception of ultrasound waves. This is accomplished by two dedicated transducer elements: one that solely sends a signal and another that only receives. With continuous-wave Doppler ultrasound, the emitting and receiving crystals function continuously and display information representative of all moving targets in the ultrasound beam. The continuous mode has no limitation of recordable velocities and therefore allows accurate measurement of high velocities. The signal, however, is not gated (it receives all underlying velocities); thus, spatial localization of the abnormal velocities is lacking. (Currie et al.)

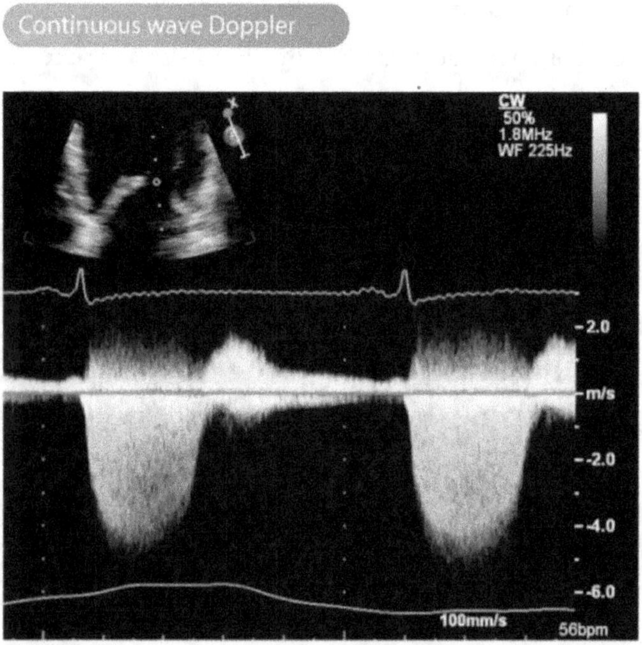

Figure 4: Continuous Wave Doppler

Image link: https://ecgwaves.com/wp-content/uploads/2019/11/continuous-wave-doppler-cw-ultrasound-echocardiography.jpg

Duplex ultrasound:

Duplex <u>ultrasound</u> is a test to see how blood moves through your arteries and veins. It records sound waves reflecting off moving objects, such as blood, to measure their speed and other aspects of how they flow. (Armstrong et al.)

There are different types of duplex ultrasound exams. Some include:

- Arterial and venous duplex ultrasound of the abdomen. This test examines blood vessels and blood flow in the abdominal area.

- Carotid duplex ultrasound looks at the carotid artery in the neck.

- Duplex ultrasound of the extremities looks at the arms or legs.

- Renal duplex ultrasound examines the kidneys and their blood vessels

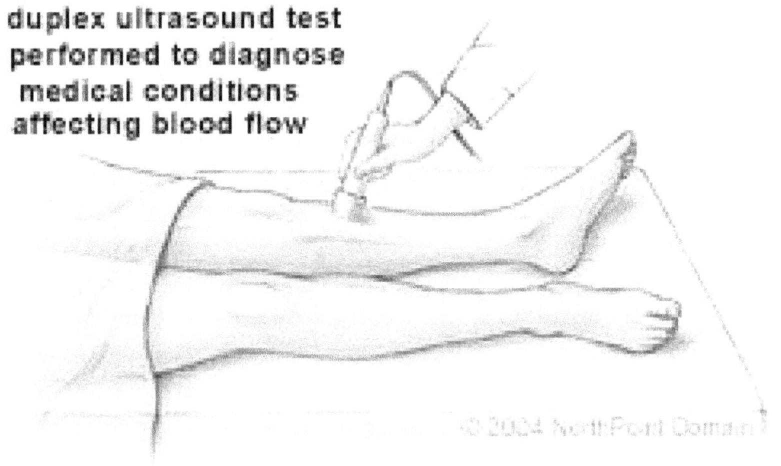

Figure 5a)

Image link: <u>http://www.rad-inc.com/images/dynamic/ACF16EC.jpg</u>

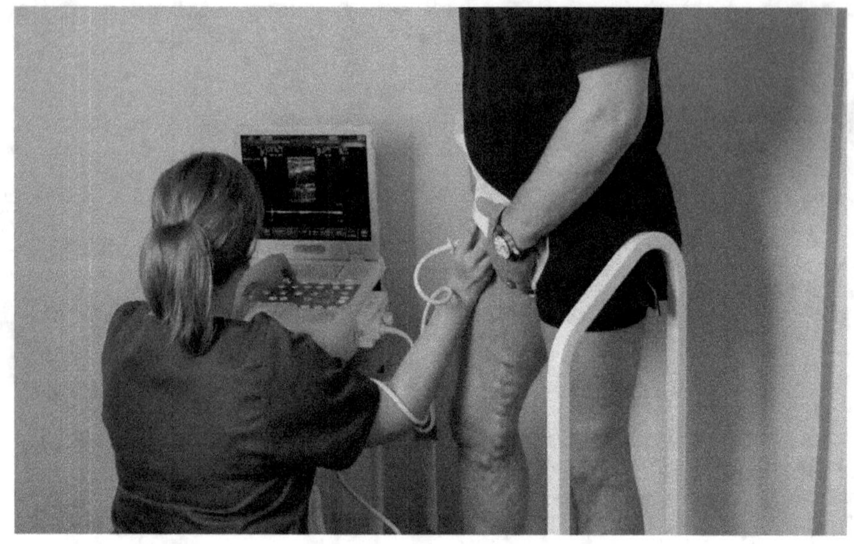

Figure 5 b)

Image link: https://images-na.ssl-images-amazon.com/images/S/videodirect-images/hero/ba55b2f0-22af-1a06-fff6-0ef5b7c461e9._SX1080_.png

1. What is the role of compression therapy in the treatment of venous disease?

Compression therapy is the cornerstone of the treatment of venous edema and lymphatic disorders. Compression therapy decreases the foot and leg volume and reduces venous reflux and venous hypertension. Medical compression therapy includes garments or devices that provide static or dynamic mechanical compression to a body region. For the treatment of lower extremity chronic venous insufficiency, static compression includes compression hosiery and compression bandages. Dynamic (intermittent) compression therapy in the form of intermittent pneumatic compression pumps and sleeves may be useful under select circumstances. For patients with venous ulceration, the benefits of long-term compression therapy (stockings or bandages) have repeatedly been demonstrated in randomized trials. (Palfreyman, Lochiel and Michaels) Healing rates as high as 97 percent can be achieved in those who are compliant with therapy. Patients with edema, weeping, or skin changes in the absence of ulceration also benefit. The goals of treatment are ulcer healing and reduction of the extent of edema, lipodermatosclerosis, and pain.

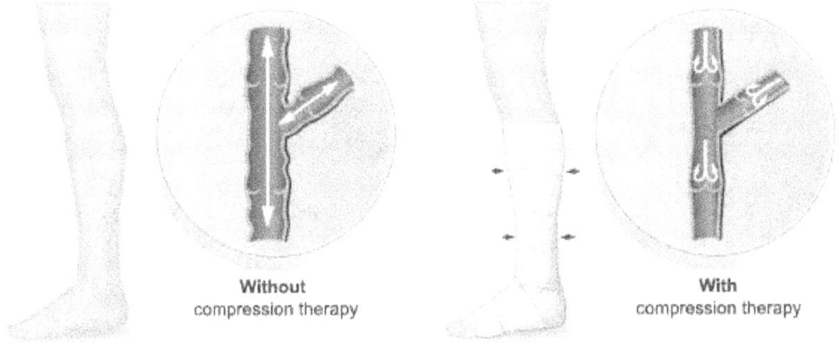

Figure 6

Image link: http://www.urgo.co.uk/uploaded-files/img/images/compression3-graph-03-petit2.jpg

2. What is the incidence, prevalence, morbidity, and comorbidity of obesity worldwide?

Incidence & Prevalence

Some recent WHO global estimates follow.

- In 2016, more than 1.9 billion adults aged 18 years and older were overweight. Of these over 650 million adults were obese.

- In 2016, 39% of adults aged 18 years and over (39% of men and 40% of women) were overweight.

- Overall, about 13% of the world's adult population (11% of men and 15% of women) were obese in 2016.

- The worldwide prevalence of obesity nearly tripled between 1975 and 2016.

- Over 340 million children and adolescents aged 5-19 were overweight or obese in 2016.

- The prevalence of overweight and obesity among children and adolescents aged 5-19 has risen dramatically from just 4% in 1975 to just over 18% in 2016. The rise has occurred similarly among both boys and girls: in 2016 18% of girls and 19% of boys were overweight.

- While just under 1% of children and adolescents aged 5-19 were obese in 1975, more 124 million children and adolescents (6% of girls and 8% of boys) were obese in 2016. (Arroyo-Johnson and Mincey)

In 2016, an estimated 41 million children under the age of 5 years were overweight or obese. Once considered a high-income country problem, overweight and obesity are now on the rise in low- and middle-income countries, particularly in urban settings. In Africa, the number of overweight children under 5 has increased by nearly 5 percent since 2000. Nearly half of the children under 5 who were overweight or obese in 2016 lived in Asia. More than half of the European population is overweight and up to 30% is obese with prevalence worldwide doubling since 1980 [World Health Organization (WHO) 2011] (Arroyo-Johnson and Mincey)

Overweight and obesity are linked to more deaths worldwide than underweight. Globally there are more people who are obese than underweight – this occurs in every region except parts of sub-Saharan Africa and Asia.

Morbidity

Obesity and its repercussions constitute an important source of morbidity, impaired quality of life and its complications can have a major bearing on life expectancy. In a meta-analysis study of 2.88 million individuals, obesity was associated with an increase in mortality rate, with a hazard ratio of 1.18 (95% CI, 1.12–1.25). (Flegal et al.) Nearly 30 percent more people worldwide died from being obese in 2015 than in 1990, according to a new study published today in the *New England Journal of Medicine*. A quarter-century ago, about 50 deaths out of every 100,000 were related to being overweight. As of 2015, the number is now 54 out of every 100,000. (Aronne)

Co-morbidities

Obesity is associated with higher rates of death driven by comorbidities such as:

- Type 2 diabetes mellitus (T2DM), The term "diabesity" is used to describe the overlap between T2DM and obesity. About 50% of diagnosed diabetic patients are obese, but only approximately 20% of patients seeking bariatric surgery are diabetic.

- Dyslipidemia: The dyslipidemia is associated with obesity leading to progressive Chronic Kidney Disease (CKD) by promoting inflammation and endothelial dysfunction. Lower concentrations of HDL, are associated with a higher incidence of CKD in the general population.

- Hypertension: Obese patients are 3.5 times more likely to have hypertension, while 60–70% of hypertension in adults may be attributable to adiposity.

- Obstructive sleep apnea (OSA): Psychosocial dysfunction, OSA, and osteoarthritis can be a direct result of increased fat mass

- <u>Certain types of cancer:</u> Cardiovascular disease (CVD) and cancer account for the greatest mortality risk associated with obesity. Obesity increases cancer incidence partly by converting a high-fat diet supplied fatty acids or *de novo* synthesized fatty acids into protumorigenic signaling lipids. Signaling lipids then signal onto the cancer cell through paracrine or autocrine interactions, while aggressive cancer cells upregulate monoacylglycerol lipase to generate fatty acids. These are incorporated in oncogenic signaling lipids that in-turn drives cancer pathogenicity.

- <u>Steatohepatitis:</u> Nonalcoholic fatty liver disease (NAFLD) includes hepatic steatosis, non-alcoholic steatohepatitis (NASH), fibrosis, and cirrhosis. NAFLD is the most common cause of chronic liver disease in the United States. Obesity and insulin resistance are considered to be the main causative factors of NAFLD.

- <u>Gastroesophageal reflux:</u> The prevalence of gastroesophageal reflux disease (GERD) is estimated to be 20–44% in the Western countries, with a lower frequency in Asia. In particular, this escalation is suggested to be related to the global rise in obesity.

- Arthritis

- Polycystic ovary syndrome (PCOS), and

- <u>Infertility:</u> Fertility can be negatively affected by obesity. In women, early onset of obesity favours the development of menses irregularities, chronic oligo-anovulation and infertility in the adult age. Obesity in women can also increase the risk of miscarriages and impair the outcomes of assisted reproductive technologies and pregnancy when the body mass index exceeds 30 kg/m^2. (Pasquali, Patton and Gambineri)

- <u>CVD</u>: Obesity associated with metabolic syndrome is associated with CVD. Metabolic syndrome is defined as a combination of at least three of the following features: central obesity, high serum triglyceride (TG) levels, low serum high-density lipoprotein (HDL), cholesterol levels, hypertension, and elevated fasting blood glucose levels. Cardiomyopathy associated with obesity is characterized by left ventricular hypertrophy and diastolic dysfunction. (Owens)

3. **What is the incidence and prevalence of cellulite as an inflammatory disease of the deep dermis?**

Cellulite is an alteration in skin topography most often found on the buttocks and posterolateral thighs of the majority of postpubertal females.

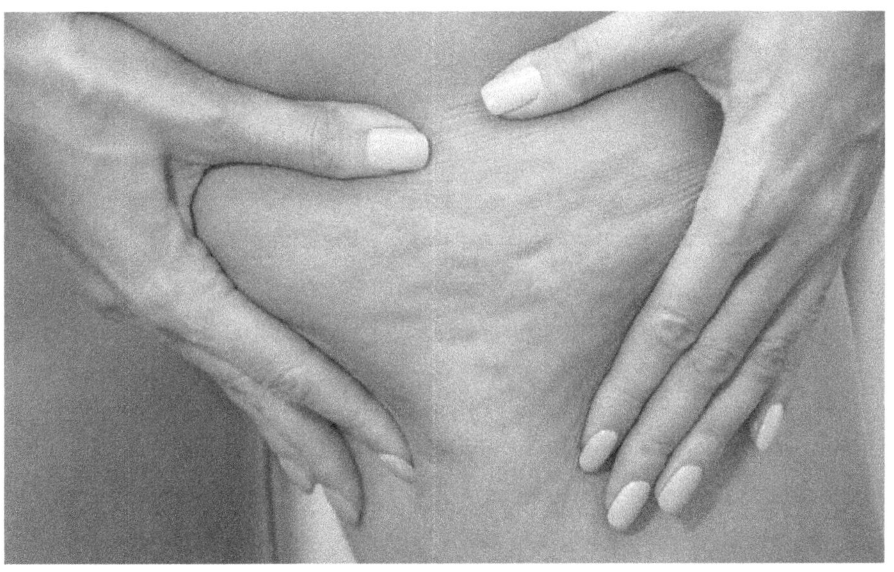

Figure 7: Cellulite

Image link: https://dcd2fe06bf58808e48f5-
f58c1372aeba1bc7277f53e7c981d121.ssl.cf5.rackcdn.com/557dffd0b1e811e8949645624205f98d_s
hutterstock_483348649.jpg

Incidence & Prevalence:

There is up to 80-90% of the prevalence of cellulite in postpubertal females. The prevalence in 2012 of cellulite was 85% amongst the 1.4 billion women aged 25-60 across the world, of whom 80% are concerned with their cellulite. Cellulite can affect both men and women, but it is more common in females, due to the different distributions of fat, muscle, and connective tissue. Between 80 and 90 percent of women may experience cellulite at some point in their lives. (Uzuncakmak, Akdeniz and Karadag)

4. How does the lymphatic system have an important role in maintaining optimal health?

The lymphatic system helps defend the body against illness-causing germs, bacteria, viruses and fungi. The system builds immunity by making special white blood cells (called lymphocytes) that produce antibodies which are responsible for immune responses that defend the body against disease. The lymphatic system is a network of tissues and organs that help rid the body of toxins, waste and other unwanted materials. The primary function of the lymphatic system is to transport lymph, a fluid containing infection-fighting white blood cells, throughout the body. The lymphatic or lymph system involves an extensive network of vessels that passes through almost all our tissues to allow for the movement of a fluid called lymph. Lymph circulates through the body in a similar way to blood. (Swartz)

There are about <u>600 lymph nodes</u> in the body. These nodes swell in response to infection, due to a build-up of lymph fluid, bacteria, or other organisms and immune system cells. The lymphatic system has an important role in maintaining optimal health as the lymphatic system plays a key role in the immune system, fluid balance, and absorption of fats and fat-soluble nutrients. The lymph vessels drain fluid from body tissues; this enables foreign material to be delivered to the lymph nodes for assessment by immune system cells.

5. What is the role of hormone imbalance, venous, and

lymphatic congestion in the pathophysiology of cellulite?

Role of hormone imbalance in the pathophysiology of cellulite

Estrogen, insulin, noradrenaline, thyroid hormones, and prolactin are part of the cellulite production process. One theory is that as estrogen in women decreases in the approach to menopause, blood flow to the connective tissue under the skin also decreases. It has been suggested that any hormonal imbalance that promotes fat gain over fat breakdowns, such as high levels of insulin, could put a person at a higher risk of developing cellulite. This theory may hold some weight, as cellulite develops after women hit puberty. It also tends to worsen during times when women are experiencing changes in estrogen levels, such as pregnancy and menopause. (Rossi and Vergnanini)

Role of lymphatic congestion in the pathophysiology of cellulite

The protein-rich lymphatic fluid serves as an excellent medium for bacteria to grow, and stagnation of the lymphatic fluid due to impaired lymph drainage with a consequent reduction in lymphatic clearance creates a state of local immune deficiency, which, in turn, can increase the risk of local cellulitis. (Hexsel and Soirefmann)

Role of venous congestion in the pathophysiology of cellulite

As well as connective tissue abnormalities, poor circulation and lymph drainage can also aggravate cellulite. Fat, or adipose tissue, is relatively rich in blood vessels. Decreased blood flow, swelling from fluid accumulation (edema), and local inflammation can aggravate the female propensity to skin looseness and hasten the development of cellulite through a domino effect. (Avram)

When small blood vessels become fragile, they leak excess fluid that accumulates in the compartments between the fat chambers. This effect increases pressure within the tissues, resulting in poor lymphatic drainage.

As the excess fluid is retained in dermal tissues, fat globules cluster together and inhibit venous return. This vascular damage results in decreased collagen synthesis and an inability to repair tissue damage, which weakens the dermis. Over time, clumps of hardened collagen contribute to the formation of fibrotic collagen bands, which become deposited around fat globules beneath the skin. The tightening of these bands causes a vicious cycle that worsens cellulite and impairs blood flow even more.6 These changes have been seen in ultrasound imaging of skin affected by cellulite, which reveals thinning of the dermis with fat pushing upward.

6. What are the medical and legal ramifications surrounding mesotherapy worldwide

Mesotherapy

It is a modern form of therapy that consists of <u>injecting</u> medicines, vitamins and minerals as close as possible to the area that needs treatment. It is an astonishingly effective technique in aesthetic medicine as it treats layers of the <u>skin</u>, which are hardly penetrated by other <u>non-invasive</u> treatments.

Mesotherapy, as a procedure, hasn't been approved by the U.S. Food and Drug Administration (FDA), but many of the ingredients used in the treatment do have FDA approval for treating other conditions. As long as the ingredients have FDA approval, they may be used for mesotherapy. This is considered to be off-label use of the approved ingredients. Practitioners don't use any standard formulas for mesotherapy. That means a person might get a completely different treatment with one doctor than you would with another. To try mesotherapy, one must see a licensed doctor who has a lot of experience with the procedure. This will help minimize side effects. (Matarasso and Pfeifer)

In America and other developed countries, as the promotion and popularity of mesotherapy and injection lipolysis have increased, so too have the questions surrounding their use. The recent FDA approval of one formulation has led to increasing levels of evidence-based studies about that product. There are also valid concerns about its off-label use. Because similar therapies remain in use, it is necessary to critically evaluate each therapy's safety and efficacy and understand the federal and state regulations surrounding each therapy's use, before pursuing mesotherapy or injection lipolysis in practice. Plastic surgeons should be aware of the medico-legal aspects associated with these therapies and the literature available on their outcomes. In 2015, DCA injection Kybella became the first FDA approved drug for "improvement of moderate to severe convexity or fullness associated with submental fat in adults.

Mesotherapy is used with consent in many countries around the world, although in some its use is under discussion because of the lack of standards, or because it is used for cosmetic purposes by non-medical personnel. The misleading advertising on injectable products should also be monitored and discouraged and continuing medical education (CME) for physicians by non-partisan organizations should be mandatory to keep up-to-date and to avoid malpractice.

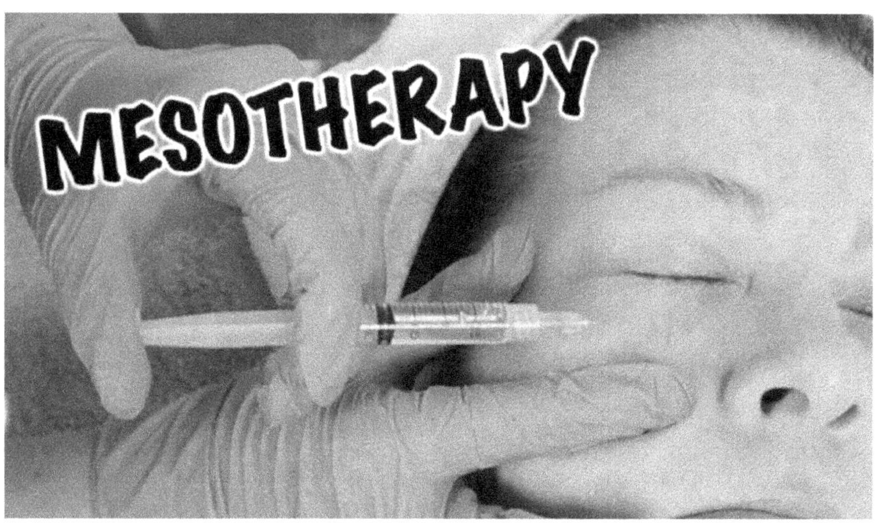

Figure 8

Image link: https://i.ytimg.com/vi/S-egmiruhvc/maxresdefault.jpg

4. **What are the energy-based devices used to treat obesity, localized adiposity, cellulite, and skin laxity including vacuum massage, infrared light, light-emitting diodes (LED), radiofrequency, and acoustic wave technology with their appropriate indications and expected clinical outcomes?**

<u>Vacuum Therapy:</u> Vacuum massage is a non-invasive mechanical massage technique performed with a mechanical device that lifts the skin through suction, creates a skin fold and mobilizes that skin fold. In the late 1970s, this therapy was introduced to treat traumatic or burn scars.

✓ Weight loss: The vacuum creates a low atmospheric pressure, increasing the blood supply and circulation to the cellulite and fat prone areas of the lower body. Thanks to this increase in blood circulation, fats can be transported from fat cells into the working muscles where they can be burnt off. This increased supply of blood, nutrition and oxygen to the lower body, while exercising the muscles, results in higher metabolism, cell activity and faster fat burning.

✓ Cellulite reduction: The sub-atmospheric pressure, created by the vacuum, not only activates the metabolism of fats, but also the lymphatic system, which ensures better removal of metabolic waste products. Stronger blood circulation to the skin and an enriched supply of oxygen, vitamins, minerals and enzymes act positively against orange peel skin. Long-term studies on women with a predisposition to cellulite and fat have not only shown the durability of the results achieved from vacuum therapy but, as an added bonus in many cases, formative tissue in the affected areas has regenerated- turning back the skin's biological clock by up to 10 years.

✓ Skin laxity: Using high-frequency Radio Frequency and vacuum technology combined, direct access is significantly increased to the deeper fat cells, bringing fat cells to a fast-active state from the production of localised heat, so that effective blood circulation occurs. This increased localised blood circulation within the dermis aims to tighten the sagging or loose skin due to the normal effects of ageing.

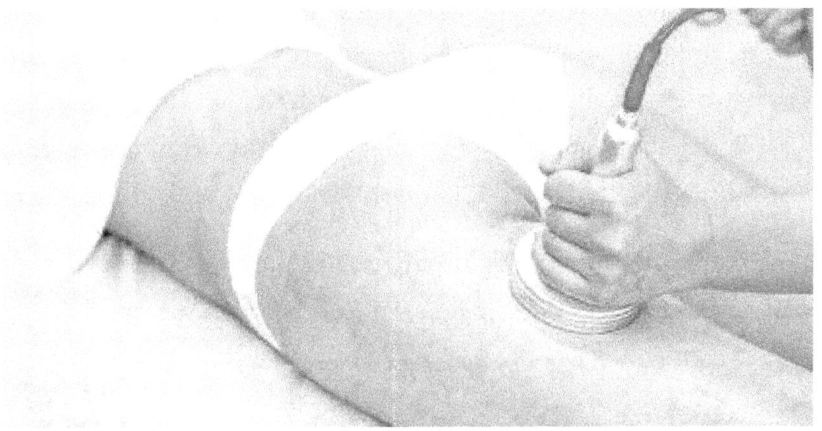

Figure 9: Vacuum massage

Image link: https://www.mybenta.com/img/8826205.jpg

Infrared light: Infrared light is defined as light penetrating wavelengths between 850nm – 1750nm.

✓ Weight loss: The concentrated wavelengths of therapeutic natural light to the skin and cells, where it reduces oxidative stress and **stimulates cellular energy production** (adenosine triphosphate or ATP). Not only does that help the body power itself more effectively, but researchers believe red light therapy affects adipocytes, which are cells that store fat, causing the lipids to disperse. In other words, light therapy helps the body wash away fat cells.

✓ Cellulite reduction: In a 2011 study on red light therapy and cellulite reduction, women ages 25-55 were divided into two groups: some did treadmill exercise + red light therapy twice a week, while the other group just did treadmill exercise. The researchers presented thermographic photographs of the changes in thigh circumference and cellulite to demonstrate that red light therapy and exercise was more effective than just exercise alone. The study concluded that treadmill exercise and red light therapy in conjunction can improve body aesthetics. Paolillo FR, Borghi-Silva A, et al. New treatment of cellulite with infrared-LED illumination applied during high-intensity treadmill training. J Cosmet Laser Ther. 2011 Aug;13(4):166-71

✓ Skin laxity: Infrared light only gets to the deeper layer of the skin and thus leaves the upper surface of the skin unaffected.

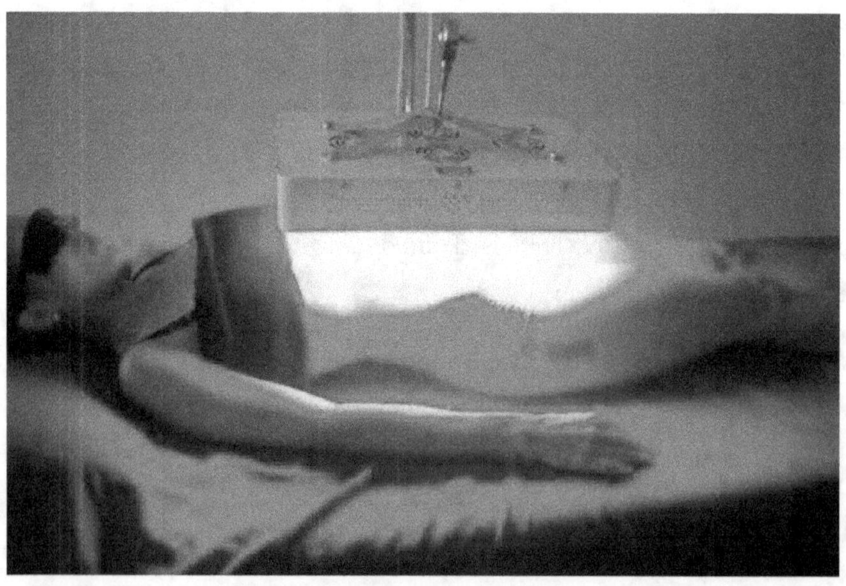

Figure 10: Infrared Light

Image link: https://redlightman.com/wp-content/uploads/2015/09/red-light-therapy-stomach.jpg

Light Emitting Diode:

- ✓ Weight loss: Research has discovered that red light waves in the 635nm range cause fat cells to dump their contents. After8 minutes exposure to red light, fat cells empty. The released waste enters the interstitial layers where they can be naturally metabolized by the body and flushed out. Red light therapy in the waves we use in our slimming and detoxifying wrap- 635nm, and 850nm waves which help boost the body's ability to process and release the expelled fats. LED can boost lymph system activity to benefit weight loss.

- ✓ Cellulite reduction: LED helps with the reduction of the appearance of cellulite.

- ✓ Skin: LED helps with increased collagen formation for skin rejuvenation and increased skin radiance and skin elasticity.

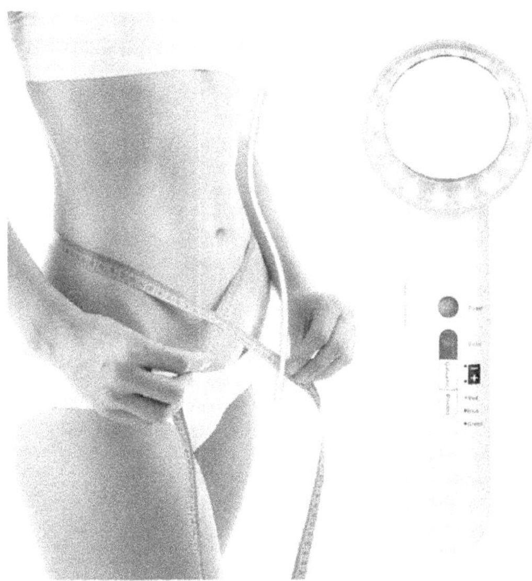

Figure 11: Light Emitting Diode (LED)

Image link: https://ae01.alicdn.com/kf/HTB1eiKSbrus3KVjSZKbq6xqkFXaI/7-In-1-RF-Ultrasonic-Cavitation-LED-Photon-EMS-Body-Skin-Slimming-Massager-Anti-Cellulite-Massage.jpg

<u>Acoustic Wave technology:</u>

- ✓ Cellulite and Skin tightening: Acoustic wave therapy (AWT) sends low-energy shock waves through cellulite-affected tissue. It's thought that this may help increase blood flow, reduce fluid retention and break down fat. Some studies have found AWT to be effective at reducing the appearance of cellulite. It was during a treatment process for female athletes that the improvements in cellulite appearance were discovered by accident. A number of female athletes were undergoing treatment for torn and strained hamstrings with Acoustic Wave Therapy with the D-Actor equipment and despite the original complaint being successfully resolved the patients kept returning for further treatment, it was during these follow-up sessions that it is was revealed to the practitioner that they were noticing a remarkable improvement in the appearance of cellulite and skin tightening.

- ✓ Localized adiposity: It is applied for the treatment of localized fat deposits in which high-intensity ultrasound waves disrupt the cellular membrane of adipocytes by causing shear stress and inducing lipolysis.

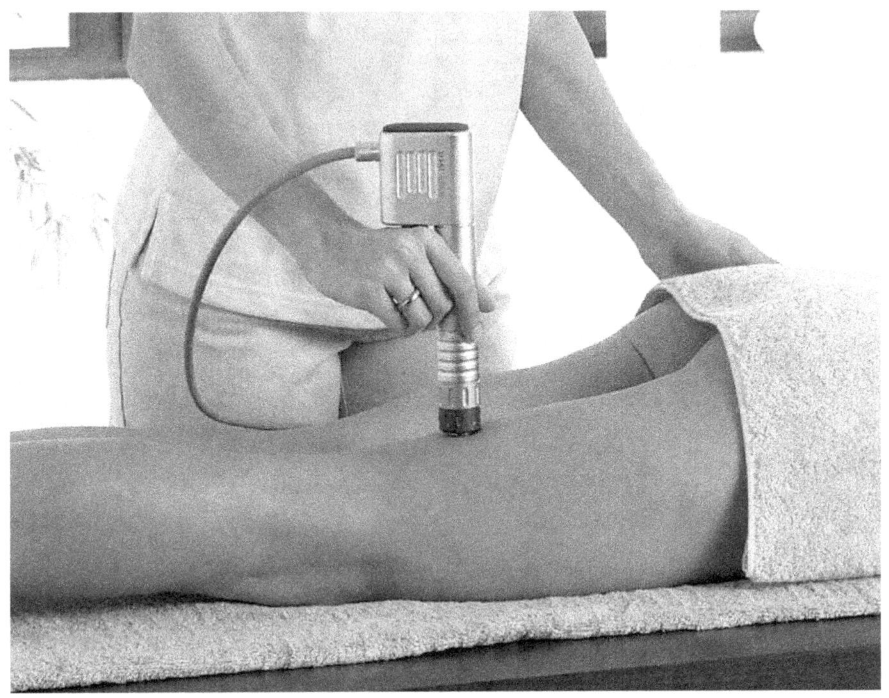

Figure 12 (a)

image link: https://www.thebodyclinic.ch/wp-content/uploads/2017/03/awt.jpg

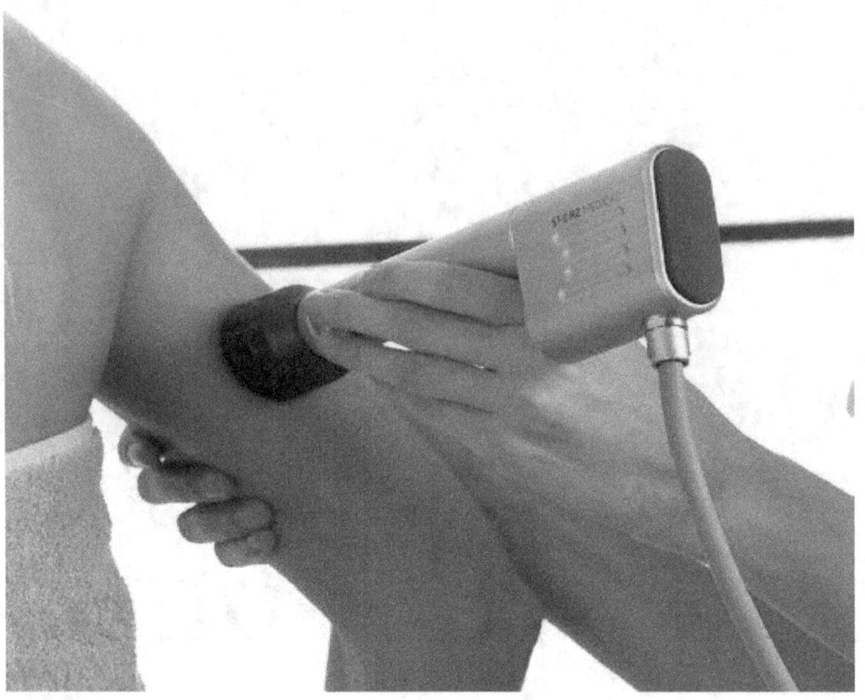

Figure 12 (b)

Image link: http://swissclinic.com.sg/wp-content/uploads/2015/12/unnamed.png

CHAPTER 21

CHOOSING A REGENERATIVE MEDICINE PROVIDER

What Should Doctors Look For When Choosing A Regenerative Medicine Provider?

Deciding to use regenerative medicine is a big decision. There are several different factors that one has to consider. Today, doctors routinely use stem cells that come from bone marrow or blood in transplant procedures to treat patients with cancer and disorders of the blood and immune system.

But according to the current scientific consensus, stem cells taken from fully developed can only turn into the type of tissue from which they came. The therapeutic potential of these adult cells is believed to be much more limited because fat stem cells can only turn into fat, liver stem cells can only turn into the liver, and so on.

Access to embryonic stem cells is federally monitored, but adult stem cells, which can be extracted from a patient's own body, are subject to relatively few federal regulations. As a result, doctors have generally been allowed to use them to treat a wide range of conditions. Thus, doctors should know how the stem cell will be extracted and make sure appropriate steps are being taken to help assure the stem cell's safety, purity, and potency.

Also, for a transplant to take place, the doctor needs to have a donor whose

tissue type matches the patient type. Matching is based on the human leukocyte antigen (HLA) tissue type. The HLA is part of what makes individual genetic characteristics.

What Is The FDA's View On Regenerative Medicine Biotech Companies?

Given the popularity and abundance of these clinics nationwide, the FDA is also taking steps to modernize regulation in the field. But despite these efforts to streamline a path to legitimacy for stem cell clinics, unregulated medical procedures persist, at times leading to patient harm.

But the Food and Drug Administration is concerned that some patients seeking cures and remedies are vulnerable to regenerative medicine treatments that are illegal and potentially harmful. And the FDA is increasing its oversight and enforcement to protect people from dishonest and unscrupulous regenerative medicine clinics while continuing to encourage innovation so that the medical industry can properly harness the potential of stem cell products.

Despite two years of increased scrutiny from the FDA, clinics continue to recruit new patients. Between February and September of 2018, these patients sought the treatments for a variety of complaints, including chronic pain, joint or back pain, rheumatoid arthritis or osteoarthritis, and rotator cuff tears. After infections tied to unapproved stem cell treatments sent 12 people to the hospital this past year, the U.S. Food and Drug Administration on Thursday issued a stern warning about the products.

Together these rapidly changing stem cell product development and regulatory pathways raise many scientific, ethical, and medical questions.

When regenerative medicine products are used in unapproved ways—or when they are processed in ways that are more than minimally manipulated, which relates to the nature and degree of processing—the

FDA may take (and has already taken) a variety of administrative and judicial actions, including criminal enforcement, depending on the violations involved.

Is There Controversy Around Stem Cell Biotech Companies?

Historically, the use of stem cells in medical research has been controversial. This is because when the therapeutic use of stem cells first came to the public's attention in the late 1990s, scientists were deriving human stem cells from embryos. Many people disagree with using human embryonic cells for medical research because extracting the stem means destroying the embryo. This creates complex issues, as people have different beliefs about what constitutes the start of human life.

For some people, life starts when a baby is born, or when an embryo develops into a fetus. Others believe that human life begins at conception, so an embryo has the same moral status and rights as a human adult or child.

The stem cell controversy is the consideration of the ethics of research involving the development, usage, and destruction of human embryos. The controversy centered on the moral implications of destroying human embryos. Many funding and research restrictions on embryonic cell research will not impact research on induced pluripotent stem cells allowing for a promising portion of the field of research to continue relatively unhindered by the ethical issues of embryonic research.

President George W. Bush had strong, pro-life religious views, and he banned funding for human stem cell research in 2001. However, President Obama's administration allowed for a partial rolling back of these research restrictions. However, by 2006, scientists had already started using pluripotent stem cells. Scientists do not derive these stem cells from embryonic stem cells. As a result, this technique does not have the same ethical concerns.

With this and other recent advances in stem cell technology, attitudes toward regenerative medicine research are slowly beginning to change.

The hope is that despite the company ultimately closing that this kind of regenerative medicine clinical science can continue as there is a huge need for new therapies for a variety of conditions including spinal cord injury and paralysis. Perhaps another company will purchase the IP here and build on some of the earlier work.

Stem cells, which are extracted from embryos when the embryos are still tiny clusters of no more than 300 cells, are generating great excitement in science because they can, in theory, grow into any of the body's cell types. So scientists hope one day to use them for replacement tissue and organs for patients with a variety of diseases, including Parkinson's and diabetes.

To realize the promise of stem cells, scientists say they need to develop cell lines that are immunologically compatible with patients. The idea behind therapeutic cloning is to create embryos that yield tailor-made stem cells, which exactly match patients' tissue.

What Is Wharton's Jelly And Why Are Stem Cells Extracted From Them Used?

Wharton s jelly is an unlimited source of stem cells that can be used in cell therapy and tissue engineering without any ethical concern. It has been revealed the cell-free extract could be effective to induce cell differentiation.

Wharton`s jelly-derived mesenchymal stem cells (WJ-MSCs), have a high proliferation valency and they do not produce teratogen or carcinogen after subsequent transplantation. They are known as regenerative medicine. Thus more research is needed on the isolation and characterization of mesenchymal stem cells.

These cells have been shown to have the desired capacity for proliferation, differentiation, and release of trophic factors that make them an excellent candidate for use in the clinical setting to provide cell- based restoration of hyaline-like cartilage.

In the current study, the researchers characterized the best way to isolate the mesenchymal stem cells from the Wharton's jelly and also compared the stem cells that come from Wharton's jelly to those that come from the bone marrow. According to their analysis, some of the critical advantages of mesenchymal stem cells deriving from Wharton's jelly rather than from bone marrow are the relative abundance of genes associated with immune system functioning, cell adhesion, and proliferation.

Each of these functions is important for regenerative medicine therapeutic applications, and so having more genes that support these functions s beneficial. The researchers also observed specific ways in which Wharton's jelly mesenchymal stem cells affect the immune system.

What Should You Look For In A Regenerative medicine Biotech Company That Offers Wharton's Jelly?

The connective tissue of the human umbilical cord, Wharton's jelly, is garnering increasing attention as a source of mesenchymal stromal cells and is now being employed in clinical trials. Also, in the public sector, parents wishing to store (bank) umbilical cord blood are increasingly being offered cord tissue, or the mesenchymal cells therein, as an additional banking service. However, there is little consensus on either how cells are extracted from the tissue or the anatomical descriptors of the tissue itself by the Biotech companies.

Conventional wisdom dictates that the human umbilical cord is a rich source of MSC. Indeed, it is the advent of MSC biology that has driven the increasing interest in umbilical cord tissue as witnessed by the increasing number of publications in the last two decades. Given the embryological derivation of the cord and the multiple mesenchymal sources that contribute to its formation, it is not surprising that some progenitor populations can be found in every region of Wharton's jelly although what is not yet clear is whether their phenotypes are equivalent.

Given the opinion that the vasculature of the cord is the predominant nutrient supply and that perivascular cells are known to migrate away from their vascular niche, it may be that the majority of MSC in Wharton's jelly originate in the perivascular region. Mesenchymal stem cells are to be isolated from Umbilical cord Wharton's Jelly obtained after normal full-term delivery. Samples will be tested for any bacterial or fungal growth as well as endotoxin and mycoplasma. The specific markers for MSCs identification will be analyzed by flow cytometry.

Today, the human umbilical cord is an increasingly popular source of cells being developed for cell therapy. The reasons, often reiterated, are the noninvasive harvest from tissue generally discarded at birth, the relatively high cell yields, and a phenotype that parallels that of mesenchymal stromal cells from other tissue sources. These cells are now being employed in human clinical trials, while also providing a cell source for an increasing number of preclinical and basic studies.

Why Do Some Doctors Choose Amniotic-Derived Stem Cells?

The advancements in stem cell therapies available in the United States are already groundbreaking, and the potential is limitless. But when such good news comes fast, it can be difficult for many people to keep up and sort truth from fiction. This is especially true regarding the pros and cons of amniotic regenerative medicines, bone marrow regenerative medicines, and adipose-derived stem cells (regenerative medicines from fat). Each has its place in stem cell research and therapy.

Amniotic stem cells can turn into any type of tissue found in joints including cartilage, ligament, tendon, bone or muscle. The only tissue they can't become is nerve tissue. This makes Stem Cell Therapy a "curative" treatment — once your joint is healed, it's healed for good! The oldest research to date shows that 100 percent of Stem Cell Therapy recipients were still pain-free four years later.

Amniotic stem cells are "multipotent," which means they can become a variety of tissues such as skin, cartilage, cardiac tissue, nerves, muscle, or bone. Amniotic cells are generally harvested from the umbilical cord after the mother gives birth. In the earlier days of stem cell research, amniotic cells were used to test their viability for repairing tissues and organs damaged by trauma, disease, or aging.

The cells used in amniotic stem cell therapy are obtained from the amniotic fluid that fills the protective sac that surrounds a fetus. It forms about the first few weeks after conception and remains until birth. When birthing begins, the amniotic sac bursts. You may have heard this referred to as the mother's "water" breaking.

Also, Amniotic stem cells have been used by ophthalmologists and plastic surgeons for about 20 years. The use of amniotic stem cells is well-researched, safe and effective.

Amniotic Stem Cell Therapy is the preferred type because patient rejection is extremely rare. Amniotic stem cells are "neutral" cells that have no DNA in them, meaning everyone's a match and you can't contract anything from the donor. All Amniotic stem cell donors go through a rigorous screening process, as determined by the Food and Drug Administration (FDA) and the American Association of Tissue Banks (AATB).

What Are The Advantages Of Amniotic Stem Cells Versus Wharton's Jelly-Derived Regenerative medicines?

Living in today's innovative society means that options for treating injuries, arthritis or other degenerative joint issues don't have to be limited to surgical interventions or pharmaceuticals. Also, new cutting-edge treatment options like amniotic membrane regenerative medicine injections may be used to treat patients suffering from arthritis or other joint conditions successfully.

The majority of regenerative medicines present in amniotic fluid share multiple characteristics, which suggests that they all might have a common origin. It has been confirmed that amniotic fluid contains a heterogeneous mixture of multi-potential stem cells. By demonstrating that the stem cells could differentiate from all three germ layers, but could not form teratomas (tumors) following implantation into immunodeficient mice, the heterogeneous nature by which stem cells could develop a variety of tissue was proven.

Amniotic stem cell treatment takes advantage of the body's ability to repair itself. With Amniotic Stem Cell Therapy, your doctor injects stem cells from amniotic tissues into your body. Similar to cortisone and steroid shots, stem cell injections have anti-inflammatory properties, but they offer far more benefits than those of standard injection therapies.

For clarification, this type of stem cell comes from the amniotic sac – not an embryo. While ethical debates have arisen about embryonic stem cell therapy, most everyone agrees that the use of Amniotic Stem Cell Therapy raises no ethical or moral questions.

Also, Wharton's jelly (WJ) of the umbilical cord (UC) has been focused as a rich source of mesenchymal stem cells (MSCs), like bone marrow (BM) and adipose tissues. MSCs possess the capacity of self-renewal and multi-lineage differentiation. Despite the recent advantages in stem cell biology, surface marker antigen(s) that could represent the MSCs has not been identified.

If Choosing Amniotic-Derived Stem Cells, What Should A Doctor Look For In A Stem Cell Biotech Company?

Advances in stem cell biotechnology hold great promise in the field of tissue engineering and regenerative medicine. Of interest are marrow mesenchymal stem cells (MSCs), embryonic stem cells (ESCs), and induced pluripotent stem cells (iPSCs). Also, amniotic fluid stem cells (AFSCs) have attracted attention as a viable choice following the search for an alternative regenerative medicine source. Doctors are interested in these cells because they come from the amniotic fluid that is routinely discarded after birth.

Deciding to have a stem cell transplant is a big decision. There are a number of different factors that one has to consider. Because Stem Cell Therapy is not yet standardized, the procedures and application of Stem Cells for Spinal Cord Injury are not uniform. And by extension, not all organizations that offer Regenerative Treatments can deliver results reliably. There are even some unethical organizations that have chosen to use the trend as a means to generate profit at the expense of those in need of treatment.

This is why it's important to be very careful when looking for stem cell biotech company.

For safety reasons it's important you identify if the regenerative medicine biotech company you're planning to get your Amniotic-Derived Stem Cells is a regulated. Scamming stem cell biotech company exist, they sometimes even use animal stem cells which is not really what you want if you're treating a muscular injury, degenerative disease or even as an anti-aging treatment.

Always look for quality and transparent information on their website also look for visible verifications in the biotech company. The medical team should be qualified. Medical staff should all be certified to provide you the service you need, and in case it's required a specialist should perform the application.

Since the stem cell therapy field is relatively new for some, they tend to do clinical trials based on the research they've done. You have to be sure about if the Amniotic-Derived Stem Cells you are getting is a clinical trial or a professional service being offered.

Also, Amniotic fluid must be harvested or gathered from a consenting donor either after a scheduled C-section operation or during an amniocentesis. The amniotic fluid is then sent to an FDA approved lab where it is processed accordingly and safety checked. After processing, the fluid is cryogenically frozen and stored. Once the fluid is prepared for use, it will be thawed and injected at the point of injury.

Finally, how they are administered and the rationale behind the application of specific procedures are matters of great concern for the doctor. Doctors should be able to explain fully well how these treatments work and how they will be administered even before the patient arrives at the clinic.

CHAPTER 1

References:

Aranguren, X.L., Verfaillie, C.M. & Luttun, A. J Mol Med (2009) 87: 3. https://doi.org/10.1007/s00109-008-0394-3

Biehl, J.K. and Russell, B., 2009. Introduction to Stem Cell Therapy. Journal of Cardiovascular Nursing, 24(2), pp.98–103.

Evans, M.J. and Kaufman, M.H., 1981. Establishment in culture of pluripotential cells from mouse embryos. Nature, .

Ezzone, S.A., 2009. History of Hematopoietic Stem Cell Transplantation. Seminars in Oncology Nursing, 25(2), pp.95–99.

Herberts, C.A., Kwa, M.S.G. and Hermsen, H.P.H., 2011. Risk factors in the development of stem cell therapy. Journal of Translational Medicine, 9, pp.1–14.

Kehat, I., Kenyagin-Karsenti, D., Snir, M., Segev, H., Amit, M., Gepstein, A., Livne, E., Binah, O., Itskovitz-Eldor, J. and Gepstein, L., 2001. Human embryonic stem cells can differentiate into myocytes with structural and functional properties of cardiomyocytes. Journal of Clinical Investigation, 108(3), pp.407–414.

Martin, G.R., 1981. Isolation of a pluripotent cell line from early mouse embryos cultured in medium conditioned by teratocarcinoma stem cells. Proceedings of the National Academy of Sciences of the United States of America, 78(12), pp.7634–8.

Mcculloch, E.A., Till, J.E. and Becker, A.J., 1963. Cytological Demonstration of the Clonal Nature of Spleen Colonies Derived from Transplanted Mouse Marrow Cells. Nature, 197(4866), pp.452–454.

NIH, 2009. Stem cell: what's in a name? Nature Reports Stem Cells, 19, pp.1–26.

Perin, E.C., Geng, Y.-J. and Willerson, J.T., 2003. Adult Stem Cell Therapy in Perspective. Circulation, 107(7), pp.935–938.

Shen, M.M., Abate-Shen, C., Kregel, S., Kiriluk, K.J., Rosen, A.M., Cai, Y., Reyes, E.E., Otto, K.B., Tom, W., Paner, G.P., Szmulewitz, R.Z., Vander Griend, D.J., Parker, A.S., Thiel, D.D., Bergstralh, E., Carlson, R.E., Rangel, L.J., Joseph, R.W., Diehl, N., Karnes, R.J., Lee, S.H., Johnson, D.T., Luong, R., Sun, Z., Morgan, T.M., Koreckij, T.D., Corey, E., Lindqvist, J., Imanishi, S.Y., Torvaldson, E., Malinen, M., Remes, M., Örn, F., Palvimo, J.J., Eriksson, J.E., Kwak, M.K., Johnson, D.T., Zhu, C., Lee, S.H., Ye, D.-W., Luong, R., Sun, Z., Lin, H.-P., Lin, C.-Y., Huo, C., Jan, Y.-J., Tseng, J.-C., Jiang, S.S., Kuo, Y.-Y., Chen, S.-C., Wang, C.-T., Chan, T.-M., Liou, J.-Y., Wang, J., Chang, W.-S.W., Chang, C.-H., Kung, H.-J., Chuu, C.-P., Bjerke, G.A., Yang, C.-S., Frierson, H.F., Paschal, B.M., Wotton, D., Liu, L., Dong, X. and Epstein, Jonathan I. MD; Egevad, Lars MD, PhD; Amin, Mahul B. MD; Delahunt, Brett MD; Srigley, John R. MD; Humphrey, Peter A. MD, P. and the G.C., 2013. The 2014 International Society of Urological Pathology (ISUP) Consensus Conference on Gleason Grading of Prostatic Carcinoma: Definition of Grading Patterns and Proposal for a New Grading System. PloS one, 8(2), pp.244–252.

Thomson, J.A., 1998. Embryonic stem cell lines derived from human blastocysts. Science, 282(5391), pp.1145–1147.

CHAPTER 2

References:

1. Kim N, Cho SG. Clinical applications of mesenchymal stem cells. *Korean J Intern Med.* 2013 Jul;28(4):387-402. doi: 10.3904/kjim.2013.28.4.387. Epub 2013 Jul 1. PubMed PMID: 23864795; PubMed Central PMCID: PMC3712145.

2. Shinya Yamanaka, Induced Pluripotent Stem Cells: Past, Present, and Future. DOI 10.1016/j.stem.2012.05.005

3. Macfarlan TS, Gifford WD, Driscoll S, Lettieri K, Rowe HM, Bonanomi D, Firth A, Singer O, Trono D, Pfaff SL. Embryonic stem cell potency fluctuates with endogenous retrovirus activity. *Nature.* 2012 Jul 5;487(7405):57-63. doi: 10.1038/nature11244. PubMed PMID: 22722858; PubMed Central PMCID: PMC3395470.

4. Henig I, Zuckerman T. Hematopoietic stem cell transplantation-50 years of evolution and future perspectives. *Rambam Maimonides Med J.* 2014 Oct 29;5(4):e0028. doi: 10.5041/RMMJ.10162. PubMed PMID: 25386344; PubMed Central PMCID: PMC4222417.

5. Moreau A, Varey E, Anegon I, Cuturi MC. Effector mechanisms of rejection. *Cold Spring Harb Perspect Med.* 2013 Nov 1;3(11):a015461. doi: 10.1101/cshperspect.a015461. PubMed PMID: 24186491; PubMed Central PMCID: PMC3808773.

6. Orlando G, Soker S, Stratta RJ, Atala A. Will regenerative medicine replace transplantation? *Cold Spring Harb Perspect Med.* 2013 Aug 1;3(8):a015693. doi: 10.1101/cshperspect.a015693. PubMed PMID: 23906883; PubMed Central PMCID: PMC3721273.

7. Weiss ML, Troyer DL. Stem cells in the umbilical cord. *Stem Cell Rev.* 2006;2(2):155-62. doi: 10.1007/s12015-006-0022-y. PubMed PMID: 17237554; PubMed Central PMCID: PMC3753204.

8. Poulos J. The limited application of stem cells in medicine: a review. *Stem Cell Res Ther.* 2018 Jan 2;9(1):1. doi: 10.1186/s13287-017-0735-7. PubMed PMID: 29291747; PubMed Central PMCID: PMC5749007.

9. Wilmut Ian, Sullivan Gareth, Taylor Jane (2008) A decade of progress since the birth of Dolly. *Reproduction, Fertility and Development* **21**, 95-100.https://doi.org/10.1071/RD08216

10. Herberts CA, Kwa MS, Hermsen HP. Risk factors in the development

CHAPTER 3

References

American Pain Society. (2012). Chronic pain costs U.S. up to $635 billion, study shows. Retrieved from https://www.sciencedaily.com/releases/2012/09/120911091100.htm CDC. (2018). Prevalence of Chronic Pain and High Impact Chronic Pain Among Adults-United States 2016. Retrieved from https://www.cdc.gov/mmwr/volumes/67/wr/mm6736a2.htm

Cirino. E. Ph.D, MSN, RN, CRNA. (2017). Healthline. What causes Chronic Pain? Retrieved from https://www.healthline.com/health/chronic-pain Cvetkovska. L. (2019). Disturbmenot! 27 Chronic Pain Statistics Everyone Should Know. Retrieved from https://disturbmenot.co/chronic-pain- statistics/

Epstein. L. (2019). Investopedia. 6 Reasons Healthcare Is So Expensive in the

Retrieved from https://www.investopedia.com/articles/personal-finance/080615/6-reasons-healthcare-so-expensive-us.asp

Guertin. R. J. et al (2018). NCBI. Just how much does it cost? A cost study of chronic pain following cardiac surgery. Retrieved from https://www.ncbi.nlm.nih.gov/pmc/articles/PMC6235323/#!po=8.536 59

Herbage. P. (2019). Center for American Progress. Too Sick for Health Care.

Retrieved from

https://www.americanprogress.org/issues/healthcare/reports/2009/07/20/6453/too-sick-for-health-care/

Probasco. J. (2019). Investopedia. Why Do Healthcare Costs Keep Rising? Retrieved from https://www.investopedia.com/insurance/why-do- healthcare-costs-keep-rising/

Tozzi. J. (2019). Bloomberg. Health Insurance Costs Surpass $20,000 Per Year, Hitting a Record Retrieved from https://www.bloomberg.com/news/articles/2019-09-25/why-is-health-insurance-so-expensive-20-000-a-year-for-coverage

CHAPTER 4

References

7 Staggering Statistics About America's Opioid Epidemic. Move Forward: American Physical Therapy Association. https://www.moveforwardpt.com/resources/detail/7-staggering-statistics-about-america-s-opioid-epi

Prescription Opioids. National Institute on Drug Abuse. Jun 2019. https://www.drugabuse.gov/publications/drugfacts/prescription-opioids

Arablouei, R. Abdelfatah. A History Of Opioids In America. NPR. 4 Apr 2019. https://www.npr.org/2019/04/04/709767408/a-history-of-opioids-in-america

How drug companies used 1980 doctor's letter to usher in widespread opioids use. CBS News. 1 Jun 2017. https://www.cbsnews.com/news/drug-companies-1980-doctors-letter-widespread-opioids-use/

M. Shah, M.R. Huecker. Opioid Withdrawal. StatPearls. 4 Jun 2019. https://www.ncbi.nlm.nih.gov/books/NBK526012/

Information sheet on opioid overdose. World Health Organization. Aug 2018. https://www.who.int/substance_abuse/information-sheet/en/

The more opioids doctors prescribe, the more they get paid. Harvard T.H. Chan School of Public Health. https://www.hsph.harvard.edu/news/hsph-in-the-news/opioids-doctors-prescriptions-payments/

How opioid addiction occurs. Mayo Clinic. https://www.mayoclinic.org/diseases-conditions/prescription-drug-abuse/in-depth/how-opioid-addiction-occurs/art-20360372

Prescription Opioid Data. Centers for Disease Control and Prevention.

https://www.cdc.gov/drugoverdose/data/prescribing.html

Miron, G. Sollenberger, L. Nicolae. Overdosing on Regulation: How Government Caused the Opioid Epidemic. CATO Institute. 14 Feb 2019. https://www.cato.org/publications/policy-analysis/overdosing-regulation-how-government-caused-opioid-epidemic

M. R. Huecker, J. Marraffa. Heroin. StatPearls. 1 May 2019. https://www.ncbi.nlm.nih.gov/books/NBK441876/

R. Benyamin, A.M. Trescot, S. Datta, R. Buenaventura, R. Adlaka, N. Sehgal, S.E. Glaser, R. Vallejo. Opioid complications and side effects. U.S. National Library of Medicine. Mar 2008. https://www.ncbi.nlm.nih.gov/pubmed/18443635

Morphine: Drug Usage Statistics, United States, 2006 - 2016. ClinCalc.com. https://clincalc.com/DrugStats/Drugs/Morphine

Ending America's Opioid Crisis. Whitehouse. https://www.whitehouse.gov/opioids/

C.A. Pino, M. Covington. Prescription of opioids for acute pain in opioid naive patients. UpToDate. https://www.uptodate.com/contents/prescription-of-opioids-for-acute-pain-in-opioid-naive-patients#H341133088

A 1980 Letter on the Risk of Opioid Addiction. NEJM. https://www.nejm.org/doi/suppl/10.1056/NEJMc1700150/suppl_file/nejmc1700150_appendix.pdf

CHAPTER 9

References

Works Cited

Alfred C. Gellhorn, Jeffrey N. Katz, and Pradeep Suri. "Osteoarthritis of the spine: the facet joints." *Nature Reviews Rheumatology* (2013): 216-224.

Andrew T. Chan, Edward L. Giovannucci, Jeffrey A. Meyerhardt, Eva S. Schernhammer, Gary C. Curhan and Charles S. Fuchs. "Long-term Use of Aspirin and Nonsteroidal Anti-inflammatory Drugs and Risk of Colorectal Cancer." *Jama Network* (2005): 914-923.

Anisimov, Vladimir N., and Vladimir Kh Khavinson. ""Peptide bioregulation of aging: results and prospects." ." *Biogerontology 11.2* (2010): 139-149.

Bachmann, Gloria A., and Sandra R. Leiblum. ""The impact of hormones on menopausal sexuality: a literature review." ." *Menopause 11.1* (2004): 120-130.

Badley EM, Wang PP. "Arthritis and the aging population: projections of arthritis prevalence in Canada 1991 to 2031." *The Journal of Rheumatology* (1998): 138-144. Baig, Mohammad Hassan, et al. " "Peptide based therapeutics and their use for the treatment of neurodegenerative and other diseases." ." *Biomedicine & Pharmacotherapy 103* (2018): 574-581.

Bartolozzi A, Andreychik D, Ahmad S. "Determinants of outcome in the treatment of rotator cuff disease." *Clin Orthop, vol 308* (1994): 90-97.

BERMAN, RAYANNE S., ROBERT S. EPSTEIN, and EVA G. LYDICK.

""Compliance of women in taking estrogen replacement therapy." ." *Journal of Women's Health 5.3* (1996): 213-220.

Binder, Allan I. "Cervical spondylosis and neck pain." *BMJ* (2007): 334:527.

Bogduk, Nikolai. "The anatomy and pathophysiology of neck pain." *Physical Medicine and Rehabilitation Clinics of North America* (2003): 455-472.

Bourke, Liam, et al. ""Lifestyle intervention in men with advanced prostate cancer receiving androgen suppression therapy: a feasibility study." ." *Cancer Epidemiology and Prevention Biomarkers 20.4* (2011): 647-657.

Busby, Robert W., et al. "Pharmacologic properties, metabolism, and disposition of linaclotide, a novel therapeutic peptide approved for the treatment of irritable bowel syndrome with constipation and chronic idiopathic constipation."." *Journal of Pharmacology and Experimental Therapeutics 344.1* (2013): 196-206.

Center, University of Maryland Medical. *Complications of Spine Surgery*. 2019.

https://www.umms.org/ummc/health-services/orthopedics/services/spine/patient-guides/complications-spine-surgery. 3 August 2019.

Chakrabarti, Subhadeep, Snigdha Guha, and Kaustav Majumder. ". "Food-derived bioactive peptides in human health: Challenges and opportunities."." *Nutrients 10.11* (2018): 1738.

Cheer, Susan M., et al. ""Goserelin." ." *Drugs 65.18* (2005): 2639-2655. Christopher M. Bono, Gary Ghiselli, Thomas J. Gilbert, D. Scott Kreiner, Charles Reitman, Jeffrey Summers, Jamie Baisden, John Easa, Robert Fernand, Tim Lamer, Paul Matz, Dan Mazanec, Daniel K. Resnick, William O. Shaffer, Anil Sharma and Reuben Timmons. *Diagnosis and Treatment of Cervical Radiculopathy from Degenerative Disorders*. USA: North American Spine Society, 2010.

Cicero, Arrigo FG, Federica Fogacci, and Alessandro Colletti. " "Potential role of bioactive peptides in prevention and treatment of chronic diseases: a narrative review." ." *British journal of pharmacology 174.11* (2017): 1378-1394.

Crofford, Leslie J. "Adverse effects of chronic opioid therapy for chronic musculoskeletal pain." *Nature Reviews Rheumatology* (2010): 191-197.

de Menis, Ernesto, Domenico Billeci, and Elisabetta Marton. ""Uneventful pregnancy in an acromegalic patient treated with slow-release lanreotide: a case report." ." *The Journal of Clinical Endocrinology & Metabolism 84.4* (1999): 1489-1489. Duman, Iltekin, et al. ""Assessment of the efficacy of gabapentin in carpal tunnel syndrome."." *CR: Journal of Clinical Rheumatology 14.3 (* (2008): 175-177.

Enbäck, J., and P. Laakkonen. ""Tumour-homing peptides: tools for targeting, imaging and destruction." ." (2007): 780-783.

Foundation, Arthrits. *Arthrits Foundation.* 2019. 3 August 2019.

<https://www.arthritis.org/living-with-arthritis/treatments/plan/arthritis-medication-options.php>.

Fradet, Vincent, et al. ""Dietary omega-3 fatty acids, cyclooxygenase-2 genetic variation, and aggressive prostate cancer risk." ." *Clinical Cancer Research 15.7* (2009): 2559-2566.

Fu, Yu, et al. ""Exploration of collagen recovered from animal by-products as a precursor of bioactive peptides: Successes and challenges." ." *Critical reviews in food science and nutrition 59.13* (2019): 2011-2027.

Gam AN, Schydlowsky P, Rossel, et al. "Treatment of 'frozen shoulder' with distension and glucorticoid compared with glucorticoid alone." *A randomised*

controlled trial, vol 27 (1998): 425-430.

Garber, Alan J. " "Long-acting glucagon-like peptide 1 receptor agonists: a review of their efficacy and tolerability."." *Diabetes care 34.Supplement 2* (2011): S279-S284. Geijsen, Niels, and D. Leanne Jones. ""Seminal discoveries in regenerative medicine: contributions of the male germ line to understanding pluripotency." ." *Human molecular genetics 17.R1* (2008): R16-R22.

George J. Christ, Justin M. Saul, Mark E. Furth, and Karl-Erik Andersson. "The Pharmacology of Regenerative Medicine." *pharmacological Reviews* (2013): 1091-1133.

Gerritsen AA, de Krom MC, Struijs MA, et al. "Conservative treatment options for carpal tunnel syndrome: a systematic review of randomised controlled trials." *J Neurol, vol, 249* (2002): 272-280.

Goodale, Travis, et al. ""Testosterone and the Heart." ." *Methodist DeBakey cardiovascular journal 13.2* (2017): 68.

Grady, Deborah, et al. ". "Hormone therapy to prevent disease and prolong life in postmenopausal women." ." *Annals of internal medicine 117.12* (1992): 1016-1037. Graziottin, Alessandra. ""Sexual pain disorders: dyspareunia and vaginismus."." *International Society of Sexual Medicine Standard Committee Book, Standard Practice in Sexual Medicine* (2006): 342-350.

Green S, Buchbinder R, Barnsley L, et al. "Non-steroidal anti-inflammatory drugs (NSAIDs) for treating lateral elbow pain in adults." *Cochrane Database Syst Rev, vol. 2* (2002): pg. CD003686.

H., Giele. "Evidence-based treatment of carpal tunnel syndrome." *Curr Orthop vol. 15* (2001): 249-255.

Harraan, Denham. ""Aging: a theory based on free radical and radiation chemistry." ." ((1955)).

Hay EM, Paterson SM, Lewis M, et al. "Pragmatic randomised controlled trial of local corticosteroid injection and naproxen for treatment of lateral epicondylitis of elbow in primary care." *Br Med J, vol,319* (1999): 964-968.

Health, Nobilis. "Preventing Degenerative Disc Disease." 2012.

Healthcare, Intermountain. "Anterior Cervical Discectomy and Fusion (ACDF); Fact sheet for patients and families." 2016.

Helmick, Jennifer M. Hootman and Charles G. "Projections of US prevalence of arthritis and associated activity limitations." *Arthritis and Rheumatism* (2006): 226-229.

Help, Disability Benefit. *Social Security Disability for Neck Pain.* USA: Disability Benefit Help, 2019.

Highsmith, Jason. M. *Spineuniverse.* 2019. 3 August 2019.

<https://www.spineuniverse.com/conditions/degenerative-disc/drugs-

medications-spinal-injections-degenerative-disc-disease>.

Hipkiss, Alan R. ""Accumulation of altered proteins and ageing: causes and effects."." *Experimental gerontology 41.5* (2006): 464-473.

Höhn, Annika, Jeannette König, and Tilman Grune. ""Protein oxidation in aging and the removal of oxidized proteins." " *Journal of proteomics 92.* (2013): 132-159. Hueng DY, Chung TT, Chuang WH, Hsu CP, Chou KN, Lin SC. "Biomechanical effects of cage positions and facet fixation on initial stability of the anterior lumbar interbody fusion motion segment." *Spine* (2014): 1-13.

Huisstede BM, Randsdorp MS, Coert JH, Glerum S, van Middelkoop M, Koes BW. " Carpal tunnel syndrome. Part II: effectiveness of surgical treatments - a systematic review." *Arch Phys Med Rehabil 91 (7):* (2010): 1005-1024.

Jackson, Owen Boyd and Neil. "How is risk defined in high-risk surgical patient management?" *Critical Care* (2005): 390-396.

Jendricke, Patrick, et al. " "Specific collagen peptides in combination with resistance training improve body composition and regional muscle strength in premenopausal women: A randomized controlled trial."." *Nutrients 11.4* (2019): 892.

Jewell, Tim. "ACDF surgery." 2017.

Jones Jr, Steven D., et al. ""Erythrocytosis and polycythemia secondary to testosterone replacement therapy in the aging male." ." *Sexual medicine reviews 3.2* (2015): 101-112.

Joseph L. Dieleman, Ranju Baral, Maxwell Birger, Anthony L. Bui, Anne Bulchis, Abigail Chapin, Hannah Hamavid, Cody Horst, Elizabeth K. Johnson, Jonathan Joseph, Rousel leLavado, Liya Lomsadze, Alex Reynolds and Ellen Squires,. "USSpendingonPersonalHealthCareandPublicHealth, 1996-2013." *Jama* (2019): 2627-2647.

Kalaitzidou, I., et al. ""Stress management and erectile dysfunction: a pilot comparative study." ." *Andrologia 46.6* (2014): 698-702.

Kamper SJ, Ostelo RW, Rubinstein SM, Nellensteijn JM, Peul WC, Arts MP, van Tulder MW. "Minimally invasive surgery for lumbar disc herniation: a systematic review and meta-analysis." *European Spine Journal* (2014): 1021-1043.

Kiet, Tuyen K., et al. ""Outcomes after shoulder replacement: comparison between reverse and anatomic total shoulder arthroplasty."." *Journal of shoulder and elbow surgery* 24.2 (2015): 179-185.

Leger, Brian T Swanson and Robin R. "Physical Therapy Following Anterior Cervical Discectomy and Fusion: A Study of Current Clinical Practice and Therapist Beliefs." *International Journal of Physiotherapy* (2015): 399-406.

Limouzin-Lamothe, Marie-Aline, et al. ""Quality of life after the menopause: influence of hormonal replacement therapy." ." *American journal of obstetrics and gynecology* 170.2 (1994): 618-624.

MacLusky, Neil J., and Frederick Naftolin. ""Sexual differentiation of the central nervous system." ." *Science* (1981): 1294-1303.

McAlindon, T. E., et al. ""Change in knee osteoarthritis cartilage detected by delayed gadolinium enhanced magnetic resonance imaging following treatment with collagen hydrolysate: a pilot randomized controlled trial."." *Osteoarthritis and Cartilage* 19.4 (2011): 399-405.

McCrory DC, Turner DA, Patwardhan MB, Richardson WJ. "Spinal Fusion for Treatment of Degenerative Disease Affecting the Lumbar Spine." *Technology Assessment Report* (2006).

Medicine, American Society of Reigonal Anesthesia and Pain. *Treatment options for chronic pain*. 2019. 3 August 2019. <https://www.asra.com/page/46/treatment-options-for-chronic-pain>.

MedicineNet. *Newsletter*. 2019. 2 August 2019. <https://www.medicinenet.com/neck_pain/article.htm>.

Mehta, Ranjana, et al. " "Proteasomal regulation of the hypoxic response modulates aging in C. elegans." ." *Science* 324.5931 (2009): 1196-1198.

Melicherčík, Pavel, Ondřej Nešuta, and Václav Čeřovský. " "Antimicrobial peptides for topical treatment of osteomyelitis and implant-related infections: study in the spongy bone."." *Pharmaceuticals 11.1 (2018)* (2018): 20.

Michael B. Seidman, Robert D. Vining and Stacie A. Salsbury. "Collaborative care for a patient with complex low back pain and long-term tobacco use: a case report." *Journal of Canadian Chiropractic Association* (2015): 216-225.

Mohamad Bydon, Risheng Xu, Rafael De la Garza-Ramos, Mohamed Macki, Daniel M. Sciubba, Jean-Paul Wolinsky, Timothy F. Witham, Ziya L. Gokaslan, Ali Bydon. "Adjacent segment disease after anterior cervical discectomy and fusion: Incidence and clinical outcomes of patients requiring anterior versus

posterior repeat cervical fusion." *Surgical Neurology International* (2014). Morgentaler, Abraham. ""Testosterone and prostate cancer: an historical perspective on a modern myth." ." *European urology 50.5* (2006): 935-939.

Nilsdotter, Anna, and Ann Bremander. ""Measures of hip function and symptoms: Harris Hip Score (HHS), Hip Disability and Osteoarthritis Outcome Score (HOOS), Oxford Hip Score (OHS), Lequesne Index of Severity for Osteoarthritis of the Hip (LISOH), and American Academy of Orthopedic Surgeons (." *Arthritis care & research 63.S11* (2011): S200-S207.

Nordqvist, By Christian. "All about degenerative disc disease." Newsletter. 2018. O'Dowd, J. K. "Basic principles of management for cervical spine trauma." *European Spine Journal* (2010): 18-22.

OjIKE, Nwakile I., et al. ""Venous thromboembolism in shoulder surgery: a systematic review."." *Acta Orthop Belg 77.3* (2011): 281-9.

Pfalzgraff, Anja, Klaus Brandenburg, and Günther Weindl. ""Antimicrobial peptides and their therapeutic potential for bacterial skin infections and wounds."." *Frontiers in pharmacology 9* (2018): 281.

Proksch, E., et al. ""Oral supplementation of specific collagen peptides has beneficial effects on human skin physiology: a double-blind, placebo-controlled study." ." *Skin pharmacology and physiology 27.1* (2014): 47-55.

Qin, Li-Qiang, et al. " "Milk consumption is a risk factor for prostate cancer: meta-analysis of case-control studies."." *Nutrition and cancer 48.1* (2004): 22-27.

Rafferty, John, et al. ""Peptide therapeutics and the pharmaceutical industry: barriers encountered translating from the laboratory to patients." ." *Current medicinal chemistry 23.37* (2016): 4231-4259.

Reginster, J.-Y. "The prevalence and burden of arthritis." *Rheumatology* (2002): 3-6.

Rivlin, Richard S. ""Therapy of obesity with hormones." ." *New England Journal of Medicine 292.1* (1975): 26-29.

Roland B. Walter, Filippo Milano, Theodore M. Brasky, and Emily White. "Long-Term Use of Acetaminophen, Aspirin, and Other Nonsteroidal Anti-Inflammatory Drugs and Risk of Hematologic Malignancies: Results From the Prospective Vitamins and Lifestyle (VITAL) Study." *Journal of Clinical Oncology* (2011): 2424–2431.

Saltiel, Alan R., and C. Ronald Kahn. ""Insulin signalling and the regulation of glucose and lipid metabolism." ." *Nature 414.6865* (2001): 799.

Sansone, Andrea, et al. " "Gynecomastia and hormones." ." *Endocrine 55.1* (2017): 37-44.

SergiyV.Kushchayev, TetianaGlushko, MohamedJarraya, KarlH.Schuleri, MarkC.Preul2, MichaelL.Brooksand Oleg M. Teytelboym. "ABCs of the degenerative spine." *Insights into Imaging* (2018): 235-274.

Sierra, Rafael J., Robert T. Trousdale, and Mark W. Pagnano. ""Above-the-knee amputation after a total knee replacement: prevalence, etiology, and functional outcome."." *JBJS 85.6 (2003):* (2003): 1000-1004.

Smidt N, van der Windt DAWM, Assendelft WJJ, et al. "Corticosteroid injections, physiotherapy, or a wait-and-see policy for lateral epicondylitis: a randomised controlled trial. ." *Lancet, vol 359* (2002): 657- 662.

Spangehl, Mark J., et al. ""Prospective analysis of preoperative and intraoperative investigations for the diagnosis of infection at the sites of two hundred and two revision total hip arthroplasties."." *JBJS 81.5* (1999): 672-83.

Staurt J. Fischer, Louis G. Jenis. "Cervical Radiculopathy: Surgical Treatment Options." 2019.

Steiner C, Andrews R, Barrett M, Weiss A. " HCUP Projections: Mobility/Orthopedic Procedures 2003 to 2012. 2012. HCUP Projections Report

2012-03. 2012 Sep 20. U.S." 2012.

Upton, AdrianR M., and AlanJ Mccomas. "The double crush in nerve-entrapment syndromes."." *The Lancet 302.7825* (1973): 359-362.

Van Riet, R. P., J. Sanchez-Sotelo, and B. F. Morrey. ""Failure of metal radial head replacement." *The Journal of bone and joint surgery. British volume 92.5* (2010): 661-667.

Vegt, Erik, et al. ""Renal toxicity of radiolabeled peptides and antibody fragments: mechanisms, impact on radionuclide therapy, and strategies for prevention."." *Journal of nuclear medicine 51.7* (2010): 1049-1058.

Wang, Christina, and Ronald S. Swerdloff. ""Androgen replacement therapy." ."

Annals of medicine 29.5 (1997): 365-370.

White, Christopher B., et al. ""Ninety-day mortality after shoulder arthroplasty."." *The Journal of arthroplasty 18.7* (2003): 886-888.

World, Foundation of drugs free. *Opioids and morphine derivative PIOIDS AND MORPHINE DERIVATIVES EFFECTS.* 2019. 3 August 2019.

<https://www.drugfreeworld.org/drugfacts/prescription/opioids-and-morphine-derivatives-effects.html>.

Yang, Ruiyue, et al. ". "Immunomodulatory effects of marine oligopeptide preparation from Chum Salmon (Oncorhynchus keta) in mice." ." *Food Chemistry 113.2* (2009): 464-470.

Yood, Robert A., et al. " "Compliance with pharmacologic therapy for osteoporosis." ." *Osteoporosis international 14.12* (2003): 965-968.

Zdzieblik, Denise, et al. ""Collagen peptide supplementation in combination with resistance training improves body composition and increases muscle strength in elderly sarcopenic men: a randomised controlled trial."." *British Journal of Nutrition 114.8* (2015): 1237-1245.

—. ""Corrigendum: Improvement of activity-related knee joint discomfort following supplementation of specific collagen peptides." *Applied Physiology, Nutrition, and Metabolism 42.11 (2017)* (2017): 1237-1237.

Zmuda, Joseph M., et al. ""The effect of testosterone aromatization on high-density lipoprotein cholesterol level and postheparin lipolytic activity."." *Metabolism 42.4* ((1993): .): 446-450.

CHAPTER 10

References:

Dr. Ananya Mandal, MD, et al. "What are Hormones?" New-medical (2007): What are Hormones?

Maggio, M., Basaria, S., Ceda, G. P., Ble, A., Ling, S. M., Bandinelli, S., . . . Ferrucci, L. (1970, January 01). The relationship between testosterone and molecular markers of inflammation in older men. Retrieved September 27, 2017, from https://jhu.pure.elsevier.com/en/publications/the-relationship-between-testosterone-and-molecular-markers-of-in-5

Hertoghe, T. (2006). The hormone handbook: a quick reference guide therapy for the physician; the keys to safe hormone replacement therapies; also adapted for patients who want to understand the details of their treatments. Walton-on-Thames: International Medical Books.

Differential Effects of Oral Versus Transdermal Estrogen Replacement Therapy on C-Reactive Protein in Postmenopausal Women," by Wanpen Vongpatanasin, MD, et al., Journal of the American College of Cardiology, Volume 41: 1358-1363, 2003.

CHAPTER 11

References

Works Cited

Alfred C. Gellhorn, Jeffrey N. Katz, and Pradeep Suri. "Osteoarthritis of the spine: the facet joints." *Nature Reviews Rheumatology* (2013): 216-224.

Andrew T. Chan, Edward L. Giovannucci, Jeffrey A. Meyerhardt, Eva S. Schernhammer, Gary C. Curhan and Charles S. Fuchs. "Long-term Use of Aspirin and Nonsteroidal Anti-inflammatory Drugs and Risk of Colorectal Cancer." *Jama Network* (2005): 914-923.

Anisimov, Vladimir N., and Vladimir Kh Khavinson. ""Peptide bioregulation of aging: results and prospects." ." *Biogerontology 11.2* (2010): 139-149.

Bachmann, Gloria A., and Sandra R. Leiblum. ""The impact of hormones on menopausal sexuality: a literature review." ." *Menopause 11.1* (2004): 120-130.

Badley EM, Wang PP. "Arthritis and the aging population: projections of arthritis prevalence in Canada 1991 to 2031." *The Journal of Rheumatology* (1998): 138-144. Baig, Mohammad Hassan, et al. " "Peptide based therapeutics and their use for the treatment of neurodegenerative and other diseases." ." *Biomedicine & Pharmacotherapy 103* (2018): 574-581.

Bartolozzi A, Andreychik D, Ahmad S. "Determinants of outcome in the treatment of rotator cuff disease." *Clin Orthop, vol 308* (1994): 90-97.

BERMAN, RAYANNE S., ROBERT S. EPSTEIN, and EVA G. LYDICK.

""Compliance of women in taking estrogen replacement therapy." ." *Journal of Women's Health 5.3* (1996): 213-220.

Binder, Allan I. "Cervical spondylosis and neck pain." *BMJ* (2007): 334:527.

Bogduk, Nikolai. "The anatomy and pathophysiology of neck pain." *Physical Medicine and Rehabilitation Clinics of North America* (2003): 455-472.

Bourke, Liam, et al. ""Lifestyle intervention in men with advanced prostate cancer receiving androgen suppression therapy: a feasibility study." ." *Cancer Epidemiology and Prevention Biomarkers 20.4* (2011): 647-657.

Busby, Robert W., et al. "Pharmacologic properties, metabolism, and disposition of linaclotide, a novel therapeutic peptide approved for the treatment of irritable bowel syndrome with constipation and chronic idiopathic constipation."." *Journal of Pharmacology and Experimental Therapeutics 344.1* (2013): 196-206.

Center, University of Maryland Medical. *Complications of Spine Surgery.* 2019.

https://www.umms.org/ummc/health-services/orthopedics/services/spine/patient-guides/complications-spine-surgery. 3 August 2019.

Chakrabarti, Subhadeep, Snigdha Guha, and Kaustav Majumder. ". "Food-derived bioactive peptides in human health: Challenges and opportunities."." *Nutrients 10.11* (2018): 1738.

Cheer, Susan M., et al. ""Goserelin." ." *Drugs 65.18* (2005): 2639-2655. Christopher M. Bono, Gary Ghiselli, Thomas J. Gilbert, D. Scott Kreiner, Charles Reitman, Jeffrey Summers, Jamie Baisden, John Easa, Robert Fernand, Tim Lamer, Paul Matz, Dan Mazanec, Daniel K. Resnick, William O. Shaffer, Anil Sharma and Reuben Timmons. *Diagnosis and Treatment of Cervical Radiculopathy from Degenerative Disorders.* USA: North American Spine Society, 2010.

Cicero, Arrigo FG, Federica Fogacci, and Alessandro Colletti. " "Potential role of bioactive peptides in prevention and treatment of chronic diseases: a narrative review." ." *British journal of pharmacology 174.11* (2017): 1378-1394.

Crofford, Leslie J. "Adverse effects of chronic opioid therapy for chronic musculoskeletal pain." *Nature Reviews Rheumatology* (2010): 191-197.

de Menis, Ernesto, Domenico Billeci, and Elisabetta Marton. ""Uneventful pregnancy in an acromegalic patient treated with slow-release lanreotide: a case report." ." *The Journal of Clinical Endocrinology & Metabolism 84.4* (1999): 1489-1489. Duman, Iltekin, et al. ""Assessment of the efficacy of gabapentin in carpal tunnel syndrome."." *CR: Journal of Clinical Rheumatology 14.3 (* (2008): 175-177.

Enbäck, J., and P. Laakkonen. ""Tumour-homing peptides: tools for targeting, imaging and destruction." ." (2007): 780-783.

Foundation, Arthrits. *Arthrits Foundation.* 2019. 3 August 2019.

<https://www.arthritis.org/living-with-arthritis/treatments/plan/arthritis-medication-options.php>.

Fradet, Vincent, et al. ""Dietary omega-3 fatty acids, cyclooxygenase-2 genetic variation, and aggressive prostate cancer risk." ." *Clinical Cancer Research 15.7* (2009): 2559-2566.

Fu, Yu, et al. ""Exploration of collagen recovered from animal by-products as a precursor of bioactive peptides: Successes and challenges." ." *Critical reviews in food science and nutrition 59.13* (2019): 2011-2027.

Gam AN, Schydlowsky P, Rossel, et al. "Treatment of 'frozen shoulder' with distension and glucorticoid compared with glucorticoid alone." *A randomised controlled trial, vol 27* (1998): 425-430.

Garber, Alan J. " "Long-acting glucagon-like peptide 1 receptor agonists: a review of their efficacy and tolerability."." *Diabetes care 34.Supplement 2* (2011): S279-S284. Geijsen, Niels, and D. Leanne Jones. ""Seminal discoveries in regenerative medicine: contributions of the male germ line to understanding pluripotency." ." *Human molecular genetics 17.R1* (2008): R16-R22.

George J. Christ, Justin M. Saul, Mark E. Furth, and Karl-Erik Andersson. "The Pharmacology of Regenerative Medicine." *pharmacological Reviews* (2013): 1091-1133.

Gerritsen AA, de Krom MC, Struijs MA, et al. "Conservative treatment options for carpal tunnel syndrome: a systematic review of randomised controlled trials." *J Neurol, vol, 249* (2002): 272-280.

Goodale, Travis, et al. ""Testosterone and the Heart." ." *Methodist DeBakey cardiovascular journal 13.2* (2017): 68.

Grady, Deborah, et al. ". "Hormone therapy to prevent disease and prolong life in postmenopausal women." ." *Annals of internal medicine 117.12* (1992): 1016-1037. Graziottin, Alessandra. ""Sexual pain disorders: dyspareunia and vaginismus."." *International Society of Sexual Medicine Standard Committee Book, Standard Practice in Sexual Medicine* (2006): 342-350.

Green S, Buchbinder R, Barnsley L, et al. "Non-steroidal anti-inflammatory drugs (NSAIDs) for treating lateral elbow pain in adults." *Cochrane Database Syst Rev, vol. 2* (2002): pg. CD003686.

H., Giele. "Evidence-based treatment of carpal tunnel syndrome." *Curr Orthop vol. 15* (2001): 249-255.

Harraan, Denham. ""Aging: a theory based on free radical and radiation chemistry." ." ((1955)).

Hay EM, Paterson SM, Lewis M, et al. "Pragmatic randomised controlled trial of local corticosteroid injection and naproxen for treatment of lateral epicondylitis of elbow in primary care." *Br Med J, vol,319* (1999): 964-968.

Health, Nobilis. "Preventing Degenerative Disc Disease." 2012.

Healthcare, Intermountain. "Anterior Cervical Discectomy and Fusion (ACDF); Fact sheet for patients and families." 2016.

Helmick, Jennifer M. Hootman and Charles G. "Projections of US prevalence of arthritis and associated activity limitations." *Arthritis and Rheumatism* (2006): 226-229.

Help, Disability Benefit. *Social Security Disability for Neck Pain*. USA: Disability Benefit Help, 2019.

Highsmith, Jason. M. *Spineuniverse.* 2019. 3 August 2019.

<https://www.spineuniverse.com/conditions/degenerative-disc/drugs-

medications-spinal-injections-degenerative-disc-disease>.

Hipkiss, Alan R. ""Accumulation of altered proteins and ageing: causes and effects."." *Experimental gerontology 41.5* (2006): 464-473.

Höhn, Annika, Jeannette König, and Tilman Grune. ""Protein oxidation in aging and the removal of oxidized proteins." " *Journal of proteomics 92.* (2013): 132-159. Hueng DY, Chung TT, Chuang WH, Hsu CP, Chou KN, Lin SC. "Biomechanical effects of cage positions and facet fixation on initial stability of the anterior lumbar interbody fusion motion segment." *Spine* (2014): 1-13.

Huisstede BM, Randsdorp MS, Coert JH, Glerum S, van Middelkoop M, Koes BW. " Carpal tunnel syndrome. Part II: effectiveness of surgical treatments - a systematic review." *Arch Phys Med Rehabil 91(7):* (2010): 1005-1024.

Jackson, Owen Boyd and Neil. "How is risk defined in high-risk surgical patient management?" *Critical Care* (2005): 390-396.

Jendricke, Patrick, et al. " "Specific collagen peptides in combination with resistance training improve body composition and regional muscle strength in premenopausal women: A randomized controlled trial."." *Nutrients 11.4* (2019): 892.

Jewell, Tim. "ACDF surgery." 2017.

Jones Jr, Steven D., et al. ""Erythrocytosis and polycythemia secondary to testosterone replacement therapy in the aging male." ." *Sexual medicine reviews 3.2* (2015): 101-112.

Joseph L. Dieleman, Ranju Baral, Maxwell Birger, Anthony L. Bui, Anne Bulchis, Abigail Chapin, Hannah Hamavid, Cody Horst, Elizabeth K. Johnson, Jonathan Joseph, Rousel leLavado, Liya Lomsadze, Alex Reynolds and Ellen Squires,. "USSpendingonPersonalHealthCareandPublicHealth, 1996-2013." *Jama* (2019):

2627-2647.

Kalaitzidou, I., et al. ""Stress management and erectile dysfunction: a pilot comparative study." ." *Andrologia 46.6* (2014): 698-702.

Kamper SJ, Ostelo RW, Rubinstein SM, Nellensteijn JM, Peul WC, Arts MP, van Tulder MW. "Minimally invasive surgery for lumbar disc herniation: a systematic review and meta-analysis." *European Spine Journal* (2014): 1021-1043.

Kiet, Tuyen K., et al. ""Outcomes after shoulder replacement: comparison between reverse and anatomic total shoulder arthroplasty."." *Journal of shoulder and elbow surgery 24.2* (2015): 179-185.

Leger, Brian T Swanson and Robin R. "Physical Therapy Following Anterior Cervical Discectomy and Fusion: A Study of Current Clinical Practice and Therapist Beliefs." *International Journal of Physiotherapy* (2015): 399-406.

Limouzin-Lamothe, Marie-Aline, et al. ""Quality of life after the menopause: influence of hormonal replacement therapy." ." *American journal of obstetrics and gynecology 170.2* (1994): 618-624.

MacLusky, Neil J., and Frederick Naftolin. ""Sexual differentiation of the central nervous system." ." *Science* (1981): 1294-1303.

McAlindon, T. E., et al. ""Change in knee osteoarthritis cartilage detected by delayed gadolinium enhanced magnetic resonance imaging following treatment with collagen hydrolysate: a pilot randomized controlled trial."." *Osteoarthritis and Cartilage 19.4* (2011): 399-405.

McCrory DC, Turner DA, Patwardhan MB, Richardson WJ. "Spinal Fusion for Treatment of Degenerative Disease Affecting the Lumbar Spine." *Technology Assessment Report* (2006).

Medicine, American Society of Reigonal Anesthesia and Pain. *Treatment options for chronic pain*. 2019. 3 August 2019. <https://www.asra.com/page/46/treatment-options-for-chronic-pain>.

MedicineNet. *Newsletter.* 2019. 2 August 2019. <https://www.medicinenet.com/neck_pain/article.htm>.

Mehta, Ranjana, et al. " "Proteasomal regulation of the hypoxic response modulates aging in C. elegans." ." *Science 324.5931* (2009): 1196-1198.

Melicherčík, Pavel, Ondřej Nešuta, and Václav Čeřovský. " "Antimicrobial peptides for topical treatment of osteomyelitis and implant-related infections: study in the spongy bone."." *Pharmaceuticals 11.1 (2018)* (2018): 20.

Michael B. Seidman, Robert D. Vining and Stacie A. Salsbury. "Collaborative care for a patient with complex low back pain and long-term tobacco use: a case report." *Journal of Canadian Chiropractic Association* (2015): 216-225.

Mohamad Bydon, Risheng Xu, Rafael De la Garza-Ramos, Mohamed Macki, Daniel M. Sciubba, Jean-Paul Wolinsky, Timothy F. Witham, Ziya L. Gokaslan, Ali Bydon. "Adjacent segment disease after anterior cervical discectomy and fusion: Incidence and clinical outcomes of patients requiring anterior versus

posterior repeat cervical fusion." *Surgical Neurology International* (2014). Morgentaler, Abraham. ""Testosterone and prostate cancer: an historical perspective on a modern myth." ." *European urology 50.5* (2006): 935-939.

Nilsdotter, Anna, and Ann Bremander. ""Measures of hip function and symptoms: Harris Hip Score (HHS), Hip Disability and Osteoarthritis Outcome Score (HOOS), Oxford Hip Score (OHS), Lequesne Index of Severity for Osteoarthritis of the Hip (LISOH), and American Academy of Orthopedic Surgeons (." *Arthritis care & research 63.S11* (2011): S200-S207.

Nordqvist, By Christian. "All about degenerative disc disease." Newsletter. 2018. O'Dowd, J. K. "Basic principles of management for cervical spine trauma." *European Spine Journal* (2010): 18-22.

OjIKE, Nwakile I., et al. ""Venous thromboembolism in shoulder surgery: a systematic review."." *Acta Orthop Belg 77.3* (2011): 281-9.

Pfalzgraff, Anja, Klaus Brandenburg, and Günther Weindl. ""Antimicrobial peptides and their therapeutic potential for bacterial skin infections and wounds."." *Frontiers in pharmacology 9* (2018): 281.

Proksch, E., et al. ""Oral supplementation of specific collagen peptides has beneficial effects on human skin physiology: a double-blind, placebo-controlled study." ." *Skin pharmacology and physiology 27.1* (2014): 47-55.

Qin, Li-Qiang, et al. " "Milk consumption is a risk factor for prostate cancer: meta-analysis of case-control studies."." *Nutrition and cancer 48.1* (2004): 22-27.

Rafferty, John, et al. ""Peptide therapeutics and the pharmaceutical industry: barriers encountered translating from the laboratory to patients." ." *Current medicinal chemistry 23.37* (2016): 4231-4259.

Reginster, J.-Y. "The prevalence and burden of arthritis." *Rheumatology* (2002): 3-6.

Rivlin, Richard S. ""Therapy of obesity with hormones." ." *New England Journal of Medicine 292.1* (1975): 26-29.

Roland B. Walter, Filippo Milano, Theodore M. Brasky, and Emily White. "Long-Term Use of Acetaminophen, Aspirin, and Other Nonsteroidal Anti-Inflammatory Drugs and Risk of Hematologic Malignancies: Results From the Prospective Vitamins and Lifestyle (VITAL) Study." *Journal of Clinical Oncology* (2011): 2424–2431.

Saltiel, Alan R., and C. Ronald Kahn. ""Insulin signalling and the regulation of glucose and lipid metabolism." ." *Nature 414.6865* (2001): 799.

Sansone, Andrea, et al. " "Gynecomastia and hormones." ." *Endocrine 55.1* (2017): 37-44.

SergiyV.Kushchayev, TetianaGlushko, MohamedJarraya, KarlH.Schuleri, MarkC.Preul2, MichaelL.Brooksand Oleg M. Teytelboym. "ABCs of the degenerative spine." *Insights into Imaging* (2018): 235-274.

Sierra, Rafael J., Robert T. Trousdale, and Mark W. Pagnano. ""Above-the-knee amputation after a total knee replacement: prevalence, etiology, and functional outcome."." *JBJS 85.6 (2003):* (2003): 1000-1004.

Smidt N, van der Windt DAWM, Assendelft WJJ, et al. "Corticosteroid injections, physiotherapy, or a wait-and-see policy for lateral epicondylitis: a randomised controlled trial. ." *Lancet, vol 359* (2002): 657- 662.

Spangehl, Mark J., et al. ""Prospective analysis of preoperative and intraoperative investigations for the diagnosis of infection at the sites of two hundred and two revision total hip arthroplasties."." *JBJS 81.5* (1999): 672-83.

Staurt J. Fischer, Louis G. Jenis. "Cervical Radiculopathy: Surgical Treatment Options." 2019.

Steiner C, Andrews R, Barrett M, Weiss A. " HCUP Projections: Mobility/Orthopedic Procedures 2003 to 2012. 2012. HCUP Projections Report

2012-03. 2012 Sep 20. U.S." 2012.

Upton, AdrianR M., and AlanJ Mccomas. "The double crush in nerve-entrapment syndromes."." *The Lancet 302.7825* (1973): 359-362.

Van Riet, R. P., J. Sanchez-Sotelo, and B. F. Morrey. ""Failure of metal radial head replacement." *The Journal of bone and joint surgery. British volume 92.5* (2010): 661-667.

Vegt, Erik, et al. ""Renal toxicity of radiolabeled peptides and antibody fragments: mechanisms, impact on radionuclide therapy, and strategies for prevention."." *Journal of nuclear medicine 51.7* (2010): 1049-1058.

Wang, Christina, and Ronald S. Swerdloff. ""Androgen replacement therapy." ."

Annals of medicine 29.5 (1997): 365-370.

White, Christopher B., et al. ""Ninety-day mortality after shoulder arthroplasty."." *The Journal of arthroplasty 18.7* (2003): 886-888.

World, Foundation of drugs free. *Opioids and morphine derivative PIOIDS AND MORPHINE DERIVATIVES EFFECTS*. 2019. 3 August 2019.

<https://www.drugfreeworld.org/drugfacts/prescription/opioids-and-morphine-derivatives-effects.html>.

Yang, Ruiyue, et al. ". "Immunomodulatory effects of marine oligopeptide preparation from Chum Salmon (Oncorhynchus keta) in mice." ." *Food Chemistry 113.2* (2009): 464-470.

Yood, Robert A., et al. " "Compliance with pharmacologic therapy for osteoporosis." ." *Osteoporosis international 14.12* (2003): 965-968.

Zdzieblik, Denise, et al. ""Collagen peptide supplementation in combination with resistance training improves body composition and increases muscle strength in elderly sarcopenic men: a randomised controlled trial."." *British Journal of Nutrition 114.8* (2015): 1237-1245.

—. ""Corrigendum: Improvement of activity-related knee joint discomfort following supplementation of specific collagen peptides." *Applied Physiology, Nutrition, and Metabolism 42.11 (2017)* (2017): 1237-1237.

Zmuda, Joseph M., et al. ""The effect of testosterone aromatization on high-density lipoprotein cholesterol level and postheparin lipolytic activity."." *Metabolism 42.4* ((1993): .): 446-450.

CHAPTER 13

Bibliography

Alfred C. Gellhorn, Jeffrey N. Katz, and Pradeep Suri. "Osteoarthritis of the spine: the facet joints." *Nature Reviews Rheumatology* (2013): 216-224.

Andrew T. Chan, Edward L. Giovannucci, Jeffrey A. Meyerhardt, Eva S. Schernhammer, Gary C. Curhan and Charles S. Fuchs. "Long-term Use of Aspirin and Nonsteroidal Anti-inflammatory Drugs and Risk of Colorectal Cancer." *Jama Network* (2005): 914-923.

Anisimov, Vladimir N., and Vladimir Kh Khavinson. ""Peptide bioregulation of aging: results and prospects." ." *Biogerontology 11.2* (2010): 139-149.

Bachmann, Gloria A., and Sandra R. Leiblum. ""The impact of hormones on menopausal sexuality: a literature review." ." *Menopause 11.1* (2004): 120-130.

Badley EM, Wang PP. "Arthritis and the aging population: projections of arthritis prevalence in Canada 1991 to 2031." *The Journal of Rheumatology* (1998): 138-144.

Baig, Mohammad Hassan, et al. " "Peptide based therapeutics and their use for the treatment of neurodegenerative and other diseases." ." *Biomedicine & Pharmacotherapy 103* (2018): 574-581.

Bartolozzi A, Andreychik D, Ahmad S. "Determinants of outcome in the treatment of rotator cuff disease." *Clin Orthop, vol 308* (1994): 90-97.

BERMAN, RAYANNE S., ROBERT S. EPSTEIN, and EVA G. LYDICK. ""Compliance of women in taking estrogen replacement therapy." ." *Journal of Women's Health 5.3* (1996): 213-220.

Binder, Allan I. "Cervical spondylosis and neck pain." *BMJ* (2007): 334:527.

Bogduk, Nikolai. "The anatomy and pathophysiology of neck pain." *Physical Medicine and Rehabilitation Clinics of North America* (2003): 455-472.

Bourke, Liam, et al. ""Lifestyle intervention in men with advanced prostate cancer receiving androgen suppression therapy: a feasibility study." ." *Cancer Epidemiology and Prevention Biomarkers 20.4* (2011): 647-657.

Busby, Robert W., et al. "Pharmacologic properties, metabolism, and disposition of linaclotide, a novel therapeutic peptide approved for the treatment of irritable bowel syndrome with constipation and chronic idiopathic constipation."." *Journal of Pharmacology and Experimental Therapeutics 344.1* (2013): 196-206.

Center, University of Maryland Medical. *Complications of Spine Surgery.* 2019. https://www.umms.org/ummc/health-services/orthopedics/services/spine/patient-guides/complications-spine-surgery. 3 August 2019.

Chakrabarti, Subhadeep, Snigdha Guha, and Kaustav Majumder. ". "Food-derived bioactive peptides in human health: Challenges and opportunities."." *Nutrients 10.11* (2018): 1738.

Cheer, Susan M., et al. ""Goserelin." ." *Drugs 65.18* (2005): 2639-2655.

Christopher M. Bono, Gary Ghiselli, Thomas J. Gilbert, D. Scott Kreiner, Charles Reitman, Jeffrey Summers, Jamie Baisden, John Easa, Robert Fernand, Tim Lamer, Paul Matz, Dan Mazanec, Daniel K. Resnick, William O. Shaffer, Anil Sharma and Reuben Timmons. *Diagnosis and Treatment of Cervical Radiculopathy from Degenerative Disorders.* USA: North American Spine Society, 2010.

Cicero, Arrigo FG, Federica Fogacci, and Alessandro Colletti. " "Potential role of bioactive peptides in prevention and treatment of chronic diseases: a narrative review." ." *British journal of pharmacology 174.11* (2017): 1378-1394.

Crofford, Leslie J. "Adverse effects of chronic opioid therapy for chronic musculoskeletal pain." *Nature Reviews Rheumatology* (2010): 191-197.

de Menis, Ernesto, Domenico Billeci, and Elisabetta Marton. ""Uneventful pregnancy in an acromegalic patient treated with slow-release lanreotide: a case report." ." *The Journal of Clinical Endocrinology & Metabolism 84.4* (1999): 1489-1489.

Duman, Iltekin, et al. ""Assessment of the efficacy of gabapentin in carpal tunnel syndrome."." *CR: Journal of Clinical Rheumatology 14.3 (* (2008): 175-177.

Enbäck, J., and P. Laakkonen. ""Tumour-homing peptides: tools for targeting, imaging and destruction." ." (2007): 780-783.

Foundation, Arthrits. *Arthrits Foundation.* 2019. 3 August 2019. <https://www.arthritis.org/living-with-arthritis/treatments/plan/arthritis-medication-options.php>.

Fradet, Vincent, et al. ""Dietary omega-3 fatty acids, cyclooxygenase-2 genetic variation, and aggressive prostate cancer risk." ." *Clinical Cancer Research 15.7* (2009): 2559-2566.

Fu, Yu, et al. ""Exploration of collagen recovered from animal by-products as a precursor of bioactive peptides: Successes and challenges." ." *Critical reviews in food science and nutrition 59.13* (2019): 2011-2027.

Gam AN, Schydlowsky P, Rossel, et al. "Treatment of 'frozen shoulder' with distension and glucorticoid compared with glucorticoid alone." *A randomised controlled trial, vol 27* (1998): 425-430.

Garber, Alan J. " "Long-acting glucagon-like peptide 1 receptor agonists: a review of their efficacy and tolerability."." *Diabetes care 34.Supplement 2* (2011): S279-S284.

Geijsen, Niels, and D. Leanne Jones. ""Seminal discoveries in regenerative medicine: contributions of the male germ line to understanding pluripotency." ." *Human molecular genetics 17.R1* (2008): R16-R22.

George J. Christ, Justin M. Saul, Mark E. Furth, and Karl-Erik Andersson. "The Pharmacology of Regenerative Medicine." *pharmacological Reviews* (2013): 1091-1133.

Gerritsen AA, de Krom MC, Struijs MA, et al. "Conservative treatment options for carpal tunnel syndrome: a systematic review of randomised controlled trials." *J Neurol, vol, 249* (2002): 272-280.

Goodale, Travis, et al. ""Testosterone and the Heart." ." *Methodist DeBakey cardiovascular journal 13.2* (2017): 68.

Grady, Deborah, et al. ". "Hormone therapy to prevent disease and prolong life in postmenopausal women." ." *Annals of internal medicine 117.12* (1992): 1016-1037.

Graziottin, Alessandra. ""Sexual pain disorders: dyspareunia and vaginismus."." *International Society of Sexual Medicine Standard Committee Book, Standard Practice in Sexual Medicine* (2006): 342-350.

Green S, Buchbinder R, Barnsley L, et al. "Non-steroidal anti-inflammatory drugs (NSAIDs) for treating lateral elbow pain in adults." *Cochrane Database*

Syst Rev, vol. 2 (2002): pg. CD003686.

H., Giele. "Evidence-based treatment of carpal tunnel syndrome." *Curr Orthop vol. 15* (2001): 249-255.

Harraan, Denham. ""Aging: a theory based on free radical and radiation chemistry." ."" ((1955)).

Hay EM, Paterson SM, Lewis M, et al. "Pragmatic randomised controlled trial of local corticosteroid injection and naproxen for treatment of lateral epicondylitis of elbow in primary care." *Br Med J, vol,319* (1999): 964-968.

Health, Nobilis. "Preventing Degenerative Disc Disease." 2012.

Healthcare, Intermountain. "Anterior Cervical Discectomy and Fusion (ACDF); Fact sheet for patients and families." 2016.

Helmick, Jennifer M. Hootman and Charles G. "Projections of US prevalence of arthritis and associated activity limitations." *Arthritis and Rheumatism* (2006): 226-229.

Help, Disability Benefit. *Social Security Disability for Neck Pain.* USA: Disability Benefit Help, 2019.

Highsmith, Jason. M. *Spineuniverse.* 2019. 3 August 2019. <https://www.spineuniverse.com/conditions/degenerative-disc/drugs-medications-spinal-injections-degenerative-disc-disease>.

Hipkiss, Alan R. ""Accumulation of altered proteins and ageing: causes and effects."." *Experimental gerontology 41.5* (2006): 464-473.

Höhn, Annika, Jeannette König, and Tilman Grune. ""Protein oxidation in aging and the removal of oxidized proteins." " *Journal of proteomics 92.* (2013): 132-159.

Hueng DY, Chung TT, Chuang WH, Hsu CP, Chou KN, Lin SC. "Biomechanical effects of cage positions and facet fixation on initial stability of the anterior lumbar interbody fusion motion segment." *Spine* (2014): 1-13.

Huisstede BM, Randsdorp MS, Coert JH, Glerum S, van Middelkoop M, Koes BW. " Carpal tunnel syndrome. Part II: effectiveness of surgical treatments - a systematic review." *Arch Phys Med Rehabil 91 (7):* (2010): 1005-1024.

Jackson, Owen Boyd and Neil. "How is risk defined in high-risk surgical patient management?" *Critical Care* (2005): 390-396.

Jendricke, Patrick, et al. " "Specific collagen peptides in combination with resistance training improve body composition and regional muscle strength in premenopausal women: A randomized controlled trial."." *Nutrients 11.4* (2019): 892.

Jewell, Tim. "ACDF surgery." 2017.

Jones Jr, Steven D., et al. ""Erythrocytosis and polycythemia secondary to testosterone replacement therapy in the aging male." ." *Sexual medicine reviews 3.2* (2015): 101-112.

Joseph L. Dieleman, Ranju Baral, Maxwell Birger, Anthony L. Bui, Anne Bulchis, Abigail Chapin, Hannah Hamavid, Cody Horst, Elizabeth K. Johnson, Jonathan Joseph, Rousel leLavado, Liya Lomsadze, Alex Reynolds and Ellen Squires,. "USSpendingonPersonalHealthCareandPublicHealth, 1996-2013." *Jama* (2019): 2627-2647.

Kalaitzidou, I., et al. ""Stress management and erectile dysfunction: a pilot comparative study." ." *Andrologia 46.6* (2014): 698-702.

Kamper SJ, Ostelo RW, Rubinstein SM, Nellensteijn JM, Peul WC, Arts MP, van Tulder MW. "Minimally invasive surgery for lumbar disc herniation: a systematic review and meta-analysis." *European Spine Journal* (2014): 1021-1043.

Kiet, Tuyen K., et al. ""Outcomes after shoulder replacement: comparison between reverse and anatomic total shoulder arthroplasty."." *Journal of shoulder and elbow surgery 24.2* (2015): 179-185.

Leger, Brian T Swanson and Robin R. "Physical Therapy Following Anterior Cervical Discectomy and Fusion: A Study of Current Clinical Practice and Therapist Beliefs." *International Journal of Physiotherapy* (2015): 399-406.

Limouzin-Lamothe, Marie-Aline, et al. ""Quality of life after the menopause: influence of hormonal replacement therapy." ." *American journal of obstetrics and gynecology 170.2* (1994): 618-624.

MacLusky, Neil J., and Frederick Naftolin. ""Sexual differentiation of the central nervous system." ." *Science* (1981): 1294-1303.

McAlindon, T. E., et al. ""Change in knee osteoarthritis cartilage detected by delayed gadolinium enhanced magnetic resonance imaging following treatment with collagen hydrolysate: a pilot randomized controlled trial."." *Osteoarthritis and Cartilage 19.4* (2011): 399-405.

McCrory DC, Turner DA, Patwardhan MB, Richardson WJ. "Spinal Fusion for Treatment of Degenerative Disease Affecting the Lumbar Spine." *Technology Assessment Report* (2006).

Medicine, American Society of Reigonal Anesthesia and Pain. *Treatment options for chronic pain.* 2019. 3 August 2019. <https://www.asra.com/page/46/treatment-options-for-chronic-pain>.

MedicineNet. *Newsletter.* 2019. 2 August 2019. <https://www.medicinenet.com/neck_pain/article.htm>.

Mehta, Ranjana, et al. " "Proteasomal regulation of the hypoxic response modulates aging in C. elegans." ." *Science 324.5931* (2009): 1196-1198.

Melicherčík, Pavel, Ondřej Nešuta, and Václav Čeřovský. " "Antimicrobial peptides for topical treatment of osteomyelitis and implant-related infections: study in the spongy bone."." *Pharmaceuticals 11.1 (2018)* (2018): 20.

Michael B. Seidman, Robert D. Vining and Stacie A. Salsbury. "Collaborative care for a patient with complex low back pain and long-term tobacco use: a case report." *Journal of Canadian Chiropractic Association* (2015): 216-225.

Mohamad Bydon, Risheng Xu, Rafael De la Garza-Ramos, Mohamed Macki, Daniel M. Sciubba, Jean-Paul Wolinsky, Timothy F. Witham, Ziya L. Gokaslan, Ali Bydon. "Adjacent segment disease after anterior cervical discectomy and fusion: Incidence and clinical outcomes of patients requiring anterior versus posterior repeat cervical fusion." *Surgical Neurology International* (2014).

Morgentaler, Abraham. ""Testosterone and prostate cancer: an historical perspective on a modern myth." ." *European urology 50.5* (2006): 935-939.

Nilsdotter, Anna, and Ann Bremander. ""Measures of hip function and symptoms: Harris Hip Score (HHS), Hip Disability and Osteoarthritis Outcome Score (HOOS), Oxford Hip Score (OHS), Lequesne Index of Severity for Osteoarthritis of the Hip (LISOH), and American Academy of Orthopedic Surgeons (." *Arthritis care & research 63.S11* (2011): S200-S207.

Nordqvist, By Christian. "All about degenerative disc disease." Newsletter. 2018.

O'Dowd, J. K. "Basic principles of management for cervical spine trauma." *European Spine Journal* (2010): 18-22.

OjIKE, Nwakile I., et al. ""Venous thromboembolism in shoulder surgery: a systematic review."." *Acta Orthop Belg 77.3* (2011): 281-9.

Pfalzgraff, Anja, Klaus Brandenburg, and Günther Weindl. ""Antimicrobial peptides and their therapeutic potential for bacterial skin infections and wounds."." *Frontiers in pharmacology 9* (2018): 281.

Proksch, E., et al. ""Oral supplementation of specific collagen peptides has beneficial effects on human skin physiology: a double-blind, placebo-controlled study." ." *Skin pharmacology and physiology 27.1* (2014): 47-55.

Qin, Li-Qiang, et al. " "Milk consumption is a risk factor for prostate cancer: meta-analysis of case-control studies."." *Nutrition and cancer 48.1* (2004): 22-27.

Rafferty, John, et al. ""Peptide therapeutics and the pharmaceutical industry: barriers encountered translating from the laboratory to patients." ." *Current medicinal chemistry 23.37* (2016): 4231-4259.

Reginster, J.-Y. "The prevalence and burden of arthritis." *Rheumatology* (2002): 3-6.

Rivlin, Richard S. ""Therapy of obesity with hormones." ." *New England Journal of Medicine 292.1* (1975): 26-29.

Roland B. Walter, Filippo Milano, Theodore M. Brasky, and Emily White. "Long-Term Use of Acetaminophen, Aspirin, and Other Nonsteroidal Anti-Inflammatory Drugs and Risk of Hematologic Malignancies: Results From the Prospective Vitamins and Lifestyle (VITAL) Study." *Journal of Clinical Oncology* (2011): 2424–2431.

Saltiel, Alan R., and C. Ronald Kahn. ""Insulin signalling and the regulation of glucose and lipid metabolism." ." *Nature 414.6865* (2001): 799.

Sansone, Andrea, et al. " "Gynecomastia and hormones." ." *Endocrine 55.1* (2017): 37-44.

SergiyV.Kushchayev, TetianaGlushko, MohamedJarraya, KarlH.Schuleri, MarkC.Preul2, MichaelL.Brooksand Oleg M. Teytelboym. "ABCs of the degenerative spine." *Insights into Imaging* (2018): 235-274.

Sierra, Rafael J., Robert T. Trousdale, and Mark W. Pagnano. ""Above-the-knee amputation after a total knee replacement: prevalence, etiology, and functional outcome."." *JBJS 85.6 (2003):* (2003): 1000-1004.

Smidt N, van der Windt DAWM, Assendelft WJJ, et al. "Corticosteroid injections, physiotherapy, or a wait-and-see policy for lateral epicondylitis: a randomised controlled trial. ." *Lancet, vol 359* (2002): 657- 662.

Spangehl, Mark J., et al. ""Prospective analysis of preoperative and intraoperative investigations for the diagnosis of infection at the sites of two hundred and two revision total hip arthroplasties."." *JBJS 81.5* (1999): 672-83.

Staurt J. Fischer, Louis G. Jenis. "Cervical Radiculopathy: Surgical Treatment Options." 2019.

Steiner C, Andrews R, Barrett M, Weiss A. " HCUP Projections: Mobility/Orthopedic Procedures 2003 to 2012. 2012. HCUP Projections Report # 2012-03. 2012 Sep 20. U.S." 2012.

Upton, AdrianR M., and AlanJ Mccomas. "The double crush in nerve-entrapment syndromes."." *The Lancet 302.7825* (1973): 359-362.

Van Riet, R. P., J. Sanchez-Sotelo, and B. F. Morrey. ""Failure of metal radial head replacement." *The Journal of bone and joint surgery. British volume 92.5* (2010): 661-667.

Vegt, Erik, et al. ""Renal toxicity of radiolabeled peptides and antibody fragments: mechanisms, impact on radionuclide therapy, and strategies for prevention."." *Journal of nuclear medicine 51.7* (2010): 1049-1058.

Wang, Christina, and Ronald S. Swerdloff. ""Androgen replacement therapy." ." *Annals of medicine 29.5* (1997): 365-370.

White, Christopher B., et al. ""Ninety-day mortality after shoulder arthroplasty."." *The Journal of arthroplasty 18.7* (2003): 886-888.

World, Foundation of drugs free. *Opioids and morphine derivative PIOIDS AND MORPHINE DERIVATIVES EFFECTS*. 2019. 3 August 2019. <https://www.drugfreeworld.org/drugfacts/prescription/opioids-and-morphine-derivatives-effects.html>.

CHAPTER 14

References

Andersson, GBJ. "The Epidemiology of Spinal Disorders. Frymoyer Jw the Adult Spine: Principles and Practice Philadelphia." Lippincott-Raven, 1997. Print.

ASRA. "Treatment Options for Chronic Pain." American Association of reigonal Anesthesia and Pain Medicine 2019. Web. 20 August 2019.

Badley, Elizabeth M, and Peizhong Peter Wang. "Arthritis and the Aging Population: Projections of Arthritis Prevalence in Canada 1991 to 2031." *The Journal of rheumatology* 25.1 (1998): 138-44. Print.

Balague, F, B Troussier, and JJ Salminen. "Non-Specific Low Back Pain in Children and Adolescents: Risk Factors." *European spine journal* 8.6 (1999): 429-38. Print.

Bono, Christopher M, et al. "Diagnosis and Treatment of Cervical Radiculopathy from Degenerative Disorders." *NASS Clinical Guideline* (2010). Print.

Boyd, Owen, and Neil Jackson. "Clinical Review: How Is Risk Defined in High-Risk Surgical Patient Management?" *Critical Care* (2005): 390-96. Print.

Cherry, Cecile. "Anterior Cervical Discectomy and Fusion for Cervical Disc Disease." *AORN journal* 76.6 (2002): 996-1008. Print.

Clinic, Cleveland. "Degenerative Back Conditions." *Health* 2019. Web.

Clinic, Mayo. "Back Pain." Mayo Clinic 2019. Web.

Deyo, Richard A, Michael Von Korff, and David Duhrkoop. "Opioids for Low Back Pain." *Bmj* 350 (2015): g6380. Print.

Dieleman, Joseph L, et al. "Us Spending on Personal Health Care and Public Health, 1996-2013." *Jama* 316.24 (2016): 2627-46. Print.

Drayer. "Pre/Post-Surgical." Physical Therapy Institute 2019. Web.

Eichholz, Kurt M., and Timothy C. Ryken. "Complications of Revision Spinal Surgery." *Neurosurg Focus* 15.3 (2003): 1-4. Print.

Gellhorn, Alfred C, Jeffrey N Katz, and Pradeep Suri. "Osteoarthritis of the

Spine: The Facet Joints." *Nature Reviews Rheumatology* 9.4 (2013): 216. Print.

Guo, How-Ran, et al. "Back Pain Prevalence in Us Industry and Estimates of Lost Workdays." *American journal of public health* 89.7 (1999): 1029-35. Print.

Hootman, Jennifer M, and Charles G Helmick. "Projections of Us Prevalence of Arthritis and Associated Activity Limitations." *Arthritis & Rheumatism: Official Journal of the American College of Rheumatology* 54.1 (2006): 226-29. Print.

Kamper, Steven J, et al. "Minimally Invasive Surgery for Lumbar Disc Herniation: A Systematic Review and Meta-Analysis." *European Spine Journal* 23.5 (2014): 1021-43. Print.

Katz, Jeffrey N. "Lumbar Disc Disorders and Low-Back Pain: Socioeconomic Factors and Consequences." *JBJS* 88.suppl_2 (2006): 21-24. Print.

Lights, Verneda, and Marijane Leonard. "What Is Back Pain?" Healthline 2109. Web.

McCrory, Douglas C, et al. "Spinal Fusion for Treatment of Degenerative Disease Affecting the Lumbar Spine." (2006). Print.

Nasser, Rani, et al. "Complications in Spine Surgery: A Review." *Journal of Neurosurgery: Spine* 13.2 (2010): 144-57. Print.

NINDS. "Low Back Pain Fact Sheet." National Institute of Neurological Disorder and Strokes 2019. Web.

O'Dowd, JK. "Basic Principles of Management for Cervical Spine Trauma." *European Spine Journal* 19.1 (2010): 18-22. Print.

Reginster, J-Y. "The Prevalence and Burden of Arthritis." *Rheumatology* 41.suppl_1 (2002): 3-6. Print.

Rubin, Devon I. "Epidemiology and Risk Factors for Spine Pain." *Neurologic clinics* 25.2 (2007): 353-71. Print.

State, Garden. "Chronic Back Pain Complications." Garden State Pian Control 2019. Web.

Taguchi, Toshihiko. "Low Back Pain in Young and Middle-Aged People." *Japan Medical Association Journal* 46.10 (2003): 417-23. Print.

Taimela, Simo, et al. "The Prevalence of Low Back Pain among Children and Adolescents: A Nationwide, Cohort-Based Questionnaire Survey in Finland." *Spine* 22.10 (1997): 1132-36. Print.

Ullrich, Peter. "What to Expect from Spine Surgery for Low Back Pain." Spine Health 2019. Web.

Vos, Theo, et al. "Years Lived with Disability (Ylds) for 1160 Sequelae of 289 Diseases and Injuries 1990–2010: A Systematic Analysis for the Global Burden of Disease Study 2010." *The lancet* 380.9859 (2012): 2163-96. Print.

WebMD. "Back Surgery: Pros and Cons." 2019. Web.

---. "Slideshow: A Visual Guide to Low Back Pain." (2019). Print.

---. "Tips to Help You Recover from Back Surgery." WebMD 2019. Web.

CHAPTER 15

References

Bibliography

Alfred C. Gellhorn, Jeffrey N. Katz, and Pradeep Suri. "Osteoarthritis of the spine: the facet joints." *Nature Reviews Rheumatology* (2013): 216-224.

Andrew T. Chan, Edward L. Giovannucci, Jeffrey A. Meyerhardt, Eva S. Schernhammer, Gary C. Curhan and Charles S. Fuchs. "Long-term Use of Aspirin and Nonsteroidal Anti-inflammatory Drugs and Risk of Colorectal Cancer." *Jama Network* (2005): 914-923.

Anisimov, Vladimir N., and Vladimir Kh Khavinson. ""Peptide bioregulation of aging: results and prospects." ." *Biogerontology 11.2* (2010): 139-149.

Bachmann, Gloria A., and Sandra R. Leiblum. ""The impact of hormones on menopausal sexuality: a literature review." ." *Menopause 11.1* (2004): 120-130.

Badley EM, Wang PP. "Arthritis and the aging population: projections of arthritis prevalence in Canada 1991 to 2031." *The Journal of Rheumatology* (1998): 138-144.

Baig, Mohammad Hassan, et al. " "Peptide based therapeutics and their use for the treatment of neurodegenerative and other diseases." ." *Biomedicine & Pharmacotherapy 103* (2018): 574-581.

Bartolozzi A, Andreychik D, Ahmad S. "Determinants of outcome in the treatment of rotator cuff disease." *Clin Orthop, vol 308* (1994): 90-97.

BERMAN, RAYANNE S., ROBERT S. EPSTEIN, and EVA G. LYDICK. ""Compliance of women in taking estrogen replacement therapy." ." *Journal of Women's Health 5.3* (1996): 213-220.

Binder, Allan I. "Cervical spondylosis and neck pain." *BMJ* (2007): 334:527.

Bogduk, Nikolai. "The anatomy and pathophysiology of neck pain." *Physical Medicine and Rehabilitation Clinics of North America* (2003): 455-472.

Bourke, Liam, et al. ""Lifestyle intervention in men with advanced prostate cancer receiving androgen suppression therapy: a feasibility study." ." *Cancer Epidemiology and Prevention Biomarkers 20.4* (2011): 647-657.

Busby, Robert W., et al. "Pharmacologic properties, metabolism, and disposition of linaclotide, a novel therapeutic peptide approved for the treatment of irritable bowel syndrome with constipation and chronic idiopathic constipation."." *Journal of Pharmacology and Experimental Therapeutics 344.1* (2013): 196-206.

Center, University of Maryland Medical. *Complications of Spine Surgery.* 2019. https://www.umms.org/ummc/health-services/orthopedics/services/spine/patient-guides/complications-spine-surgery. 3 August 2019.

Chakrabarti, Subhadeep, Snigdha Guha, and Kaustav Majumder. ". "Food-derived bioactive peptides in human health: Challenges and opportunities."." *Nutrients 10.11* (2018): 1738.

Cheer, Susan M., et al. ""Goserelin." ." *Drugs 65.18* (2005): 2639-2655.

Christopher M. Bono, Gary Ghiselli, Thomas J. Gilbert, D. Scott Kreiner, Charles Reitman, Jeffrey Summers, Jamie Baisden, John Easa, Robert Fernand, Tim Lamer, Paul Matz, Dan Mazanec, Daniel K. Resnick, William O. Shaffer, Anil Sharma and Reuben Timmons. *Diagnosis and Treatment of Cervical Radiculopathy from Degenerative Disorders.* USA: North American Spine Society, 2010.

Cicero, Arrigo FG, Federica Fogacci, and Alessandro Colletti. " "Potential role of bioactive peptides in prevention and treatment of chronic diseases: a narrative review." ." *British journal of pharmacology 174.11* (2017): 1378-1394.

Crofford, Leslie J. "Adverse effects of chronic opioid therapy for chronic musculoskeletal pain." *Nature Reviews Rheumatology* (2010): 191-197.

de Menis, Ernesto, Domenico Billeci, and Elisabetta Marton. ""Uneventful pregnancy in an acromegalic patient treated with slow-release lanreotide: a case report." ." *The Journal of Clinical Endocrinology & Metabolism 84.4* (1999): 1489-1489.

Duman, Iltekin, et al. ""Assessment of the efficacy of gabapentin in carpal tunnel syndrome."." *CR: Journal of Clinical Rheumatology 14.3 (* (2008): 175-177.

Enbäck, J., and P. Laakkonen. ""Tumour-homing peptides: tools for targeting, imaging and destruction." ." (2007): 780-783.

Foundation, Arthrits. *Arthrits Foundation.* 2019. 3 August 2019. <https://www.arthritis.org/living-with-arthritis/treatments/plan/arthritis-medication-options.php>.

Fradet, Vincent, et al. ""Dietary omega-3 fatty acids, cyclooxygenase-2 genetic variation, and aggressive prostate cancer risk." ." *Clinical Cancer Research 15.7* (2009): 2559-2566.

Fu, Yu, et al. ""Exploration of collagen recovered from animal by-products as a precursor of bioactive peptides: Successes and challenges." ." *Critical reviews in food science and nutrition 59.13* (2019): 2011-2027.

Gam AN, Schydlowsky P, Rossel, et al. "Treatment of 'frozen shoulder' with distension and glucorticoid compared with glucorticoid alone." *A randomised controlled trial, vol 27* (1998): 425-430.

Garber, Alan J. " "Long-acting glucagon-like peptide 1 receptor agonists: a review of their efficacy and tolerability."." *Diabetes care 34.Supplement 2* (2011): S279-S284.

Geijsen, Niels, and D. Leanne Jones. ""Seminal discoveries in regenerative medicine: contributions of the male germ line to understanding pluripotency." ." *Human molecular genetics 17.R1* (2008): R16-R22.

George J. Christ, Justin M. Saul, Mark E. Furth, and Karl-Erik Andersson. "The Pharmacology of Regenerative Medicine." *pharmacological Reviews* (2013): 1091-1133.

Gerritsen AA, de Krom MC, Struijs MA, et al. "Conservative treatment options for carpal tunnel syndrome: a systematic review of randomised controlled trials." *J Neurol, vol, 249* (2002): 272-280.

Goodale, Travis, et al. ""Testosterone and the Heart." ." *Methodist DeBakey cardiovascular journal 13.2* (2017): 68.

Grady, Deborah, et al. ". "Hormone therapy to prevent disease and prolong life in postmenopausal women." ." *Annals of internal medicine 117.12* (1992): 1016-1037.

Graziottin, Alessandra. ""Sexual pain disorders: dyspareunia and vaginismus."." *International Society of Sexual Medicine Standard Committee Book, Standard Practice in Sexual Medicine* (2006): 342-350.

Green S, Buchbinder R, Barnsley L, et al. "Non-steroidal anti-inflammatory drugs (NSAIDs) for treating lateral elbow pain in adults." *Cochrane Database Syst Rev, vol. 2* (2002): pg. CD003686.

H., Giele. "Evidence-based treatment of carpal tunnel syndrome." *Curr Orthop vol. 15* (2001): 249-255.

Harraan, Denham. ""Aging: a theory based on free radical and radiation chemistry." ." ((1955)).

Hay EM, Paterson SM, Lewis M, et al. "Pragmatic randomised controlled trial of local corticosteroid injection and naproxen for treatment of lateral epicondylitis of elbow in primary care." *Br Med J, vol,319* (1999): 964-968.

Health, Nobilis. "Preventing Degenerative Disc Disease." 2012.

Healthcare, Intermountain. "Anterior Cervical Discectomy and Fusion (ACDF); Fact sheet for patients and families." 2016.

Helmick, Jennifer M. Hootman and Charles G. "Projections of US prevalence of arthritis and associated activity limitations." *Arthritis and Rheumatism* (2006): 226-229.

Help, Disability Benefit. *Social Security Disability for Neck Pain*. USA: Disability Benefit Help, 2019.

Highsmith, Jason. M. *Spineuniverse*. 2019. 3 August 2019. <https://www.spineuniverse.com/conditions/degenerative-disc/drugs-medications-spinal-injections-degenerative-disc-disease>.

Hipkiss, Alan R. ""Accumulation of altered proteins and ageing: causes and effects."." *Experimental gerontology 41.5* (2006): 464-473.

Höhn, Annika, Jeannette König, and Tilman Grune. ""Protein oxidation in aging and the removal of oxidized proteins." *"Journal of proteomics 92.* (2013): 132-159.

Hueng DY, Chung TT, Chuang WH, Hsu CP, Chou KN, Lin SC. "Biomechanical effects of cage positions and facet fixation on initial stability of the anterior lumbar interbody fusion motion segment." *Spine* (2014): 1-13.

Huisstede BM, Randsdorp MS, Coert JH, Glerum S, van Middelkoop M, Koes BW. " Carpal tunnel syndrome. Part II: effectiveness of surgical treatments - a systematic review." *Arch Phys Med Rehabil 91(7):* (2010): 1005-1024.

Jackson, Owen Boyd and Neil. "How is risk defined in high-risk surgical patient management?" *Critical Care* (2005): 390-396.

Jendricke, Patrick, et al. " "Specific collagen peptides in combination with resistance training improve body composition and regional muscle strength in premenopausal women: A randomized controlled trial."." *Nutrients 11.4* (2019): 892.

Jewell, Tim. "ACDF surgery." 2017.

Jones Jr, Steven D., et al. ""Erythrocytosis and polycythemia secondary to testosterone replacement therapy in the aging male." ." *Sexual medicine reviews 3.2* (2015): 101-112.

Joseph L. Dieleman, Ranju Baral, Maxwell Birger, Anthony L. Bui, Anne Bulchis, Abigail Chapin, Hannah Hamavid, Cody Horst, Elizabeth K. Johnson, Jonathan Joseph, Rousel leLavado, Liya Lomsadze, Alex Reynolds and Ellen Squires,. "USSpendingonPersonalHealthCareandPublicHealth, 1996-2013." *Jama* (2019): 2627-2647.

Kalaitzidou, I., et al. ""Stress management and erectile dysfunction: a pilot comparative study." ." *Andrologia 46.6* (2014): 698-702.

Kamper SJ, Ostelo RW, Rubinstein SM, Nellensteijn JM, Peul WC, Arts MP, van Tulder MW. "Minimally invasive surgery for lumbar disc herniation: a systematic review and meta-analysis." *European Spine Journal* (2014): 1021-1043.

Kiet, Tuyen K., et al. ""Outcomes after shoulder replacement: comparison between reverse and anatomic total shoulder arthroplasty."." *Journal of shoulder and elbow surgery 24.2* (2015): 179-185.

Leger, Brian T Swanson and Robin R. "Physical Therapy Following Anterior Cervical Discectomy and Fusion: A Study of Current Clinical Practice and Therapist Beliefs." *International Journal of Physiotherapy* (2015): 399-406.

Limouzin-Lamothe, Marie-Aline, et al. ""Quality of life after the menopause: influence of hormonal replacement therapy." ." *American journal of obstetrics and gynecology 170.2* (1994): 618-624.

MacLusky, Neil J., and Frederick Naftolin. ""Sexual differentiation of the central nervous system." ." *Science* (1981): 1294-1303.

McAlindon, T. E., et al. ""Change in knee osteoarthritis cartilage detected by delayed gadolinium enhanced magnetic resonance imaging following treatment with collagen hydrolysate: a pilot randomized controlled trial."." *Osteoarthritis and Cartilage 19.4* (2011): 399-405.

McCrory DC, Turner DA, Patwardhan MB, Richardson WJ. "Spinal Fusion for Treatment of Degenerative Disease Affecting the Lumbar Spine." *Technology Assessment Report* (2006).

Medicine, American Society of Reigonal Anesthesia and Pain. *Treatment options for chronic pain*. 2019. 3 August 2019. <https://www.asra.com/page/46/treatment-options-for-chronic-pain>.

MedicineNet. *Newsletter.* 2019. 2 August 2019. <https://www.medicinenet.com/neck_pain/article.htm>.

Mehta, Ranjana, et al. " "Proteasomal regulation of the hypoxic response modulates aging in C. elegans." ." *Science 324.5931* (2009): 1196-1198.

Melicherčík, Pavel, Ondřej Nešuta, and Václav Čeřovský. " "Antimicrobial peptides for topical treatment of osteomyelitis and implant-related infections: study in the spongy bone."." *Pharmaceuticals 11.1 (2018)* (2018): 20.

Michael B. Seidman, Robert D. Vining and Stacie A. Salsbury. "Collaborative care for a patient with complex low back pain and long-term tobacco use: a case report." *Journal of Canadian Chiropractic Association* (2015): 216-225.

Mohamad Bydon, Risheng Xu, Rafael De la Garza-Ramos, Mohamed Macki, Daniel M. Sciubba, Jean-Paul Wolinsky, Timothy F. Witham, Ziya L. Gokaslan, Ali Bydon. "Adjacent segment disease after anterior cervical discectomy and fusion: Incidence and clinical outcomes of patients requiring anterior versus posterior repeat cervical fusion." *Surgical Neurology International* (2014).

Morgentaler, Abraham. ""Testosterone and prostate cancer: an historical perspective on a modern myth." ." *European urology 50.5* (2006): 935-939.

Nilsdotter, Anna, and Ann Bremander. ""Measures of hip function and symptoms: Harris Hip Score (HHS), Hip Disability and Osteoarthritis Outcome Score (HOOS), Oxford Hip Score (OHS), Lequesne Index of Severity for Osteoarthritis of the Hip (LISOH), and American Academy of Orthopedic Surgeons (." *Arthritis care & research 63.S11* (2011): S200-S207.

Nordqvist, By Christian. "All about degenerative disc disease." Newsletter. 2018.

O'Dowd, J. K. "Basic principles of management for cervical spine trauma." *European Spine Journal* (2010): 18-22.

OjIKE, Nwakile I., et al. ""Venous thromboembolism in shoulder surgery: a systematic review."." *Acta Orthop Belg 77.3* (2011): 281-9.

Pfalzgraff, Anja, Klaus Brandenburg, and Günther Weindl. ""Antimicrobial peptides and their therapeutic potential for bacterial skin infections and wounds."." *Frontiers in pharmacology 9* (2018): 281.

Proksch, E., et al. ""Oral supplementation of specific collagen peptides has beneficial effects on human skin physiology: a double-blind, placebo-controlled study." ." *Skin pharmacology and physiology 27.1* (2014): 47-55.

Qin, Li-Qiang, et al. " "Milk consumption is a risk factor for prostate cancer: meta-analysis of case-control studies."." *Nutrition and cancer 48.1* (2004): 22-27.

Rafferty, John, et al. ""Peptide therapeutics and the pharmaceutical industry: barriers encountered translating from the laboratory to patients." ." *Current medicinal chemistry 23.37* (2016): 4231-4259.

Reginster, J.-Y. "The prevalence and burden of arthritis." *Rheumatology* (2002): 3-6.

Rivlin, Richard S. ""Therapy of obesity with hormones."." *New England Journal of Medicine 292.1* (1975): 26-29.

Roland B. Walter, Filippo Milano, Theodore M. Brasky, and Emily White. "Long-Term Use of Acetaminophen, Aspirin, and Other Nonsteroidal Anti-Inflammatory Drugs and Risk of Hematologic Malignancies: Results From the Prospective Vitamins and Lifestyle (VITAL) Study." *Journal of Clinical Oncology* (2011): 2424–2431.

Saltiel, Alan R., and C. Ronald Kahn. ""Insulin signalling and the regulation of glucose and lipid metabolism."." *Nature 414.6865* (2001): 799.

Sansone, Andrea, et al. " "Gynecomastia and hormones."." *Endocrine 55.1* (2017): 37-44.

SergiyV.Kushchayev, TetianaGlushko, MohamedJarraya, KarlH.Schuleri, MarkC.Preul2, MichaelL.Brooksand Oleg M. Teytelboym. "ABCs of the degenerative spine." *Insights into Imaging* (2018): 235-274.

Sierra, Rafael J., Robert T. Trousdale, and Mark W. Pagnano. ""Above-the-knee amputation after a total knee replacement: prevalence, etiology, and functional outcome."." *JBJS 85.6 (2003):* (2003): 1000-1004.

Smidt N, van der Windt DAWM, Assendelft WJJ, et al. "Corticosteroid injections, physiotherapy, or a wait-and-see policy for lateral epicondylitis: a randomised controlled trial ." *Lancet, vol 359* (2002): 657- 662.

Spangehl, Mark J., et al. ""Prospective analysis of preoperative and intraoperative investigations for the diagnosis of infection at the sites of two hundred and two revision total hip arthroplasties."." *JBJS 81.5* (1999): 672-83.

Staurt J. Fischer, Louis G. Jenis. "Cervical Radiculopathy: Surgical Treatment Options." 2019.

Steiner C, Andrews R, Barrett M, Weiss A. " HCUP Projections: Mobility/Orthopedic Procedures 2003 to 2012. 2012. HCUP Projections Report # 2012-03. 2012 Sep 20. U.S." 2012.

Upton, AdrianR M., and AlanJ Mccomas. "The double crush in nerve-entrapment syndromes."." *The Lancet 302.7825* (1973): 359-362.

Van Riet, R. P., J. Sanchez-Sotelo, and B. F. Morrey. ""Failure of metal radial head replacement." *The Journal of bone and joint surgery. British volume 92.5* (2010): 661-667.

Vegt, Erik, et al. ""Renal toxicity of radiolabeled peptides and antibody fragments: mechanisms, impact on radionuclide therapy, and strategies for prevention."." *Journal of nuclear medicine 51.7* (2010): 1049-1058.

Wang, Christina, and Ronald S. Swerdloff. ""Androgen replacement therapy." ." *Annals of medicine 29.5* (1997): 365-370.

White, Christopher B., et al. ""Ninety-day mortality after shoulder arthroplasty."." *The Journal of arthroplasty 18.7* (2003): 886-888.

CHAPTER 16

References

- Marshall S, Tardif G, Ashworth N. 2007. Local corticosteroid injection for tarsal tunnel syndrome. Cochrane Database Syst Rev.

- Shi Q, MacDermid JC. 2011. Is surgical intervention more effective than non-surgical treatment for taral tunnel syndrome? A systematic review. J OrthopSurg Res

- Atroshi I, Flondell M, Hofer M, Ranstam J. 2013. Methylprednisolone injections for the carpal tunnel syndrome: a randomized, placebo-controlled trial.

- Cappatto R, Calkins H, Chen S, et al. 2010. Updated worldwide survey on the methods, efficacy and safety of catheter ablation for human atrial fibrillation.

- Haissaguerre M, Sanders P, Hocini M, et al. 2005. Catheter ablation of long lasting persistent atrial fibrillation: critical structures for termination. *J CardiovascElectrophysiol.*

- Nademanee K, McKenzie J, Kossar E, et al. 2004. A new approach to catheter ablation fof atrial fibrillation: mapping of the electrophysiologic substrate. *J Am CollCardiol.*

- Sudoh Y, Cahoon EE, Gerner P, Wang GK. 2003. Tricyclic antidepressants as long-acting local anesthetics. Pain.

- Joint Replacement Surgery and You. April, 2009. In *Arthritis, Musculoskeletal and Skin Disease online.*

- Leopold SS. April 2009. "Minimally invasive total knee arthroplasty for osteoarthritis". *N. Engl. J. Med.*

CHAPTER 19

References

Allemann, Inja Bogdan, and Leslie Baumann. "Hyaluronic Acid Gel (Juvéderm™) Preparations in the Treatment of Facial Wrinkles and Folds." Clinical interventions in aging 3.4 (2008): 629. Print.

Aoki, K Roger. "Pharmacology and Immunology of Botulinum Toxin Serotypes." Journal of Neurology 248.1 (2001): I3-I10. Print.

Augustin, M, et al. "Prevalence and Disease Burden of Hyperhidrosis in the Adult Population." Dermatology 227.1 (2013): 10-13. Print.

Bauman, Leslie. "Cosmoderm/Cosmoplast (Human Bioengineered Collagen) for the Aging Face." Facial plastic surgery 20.02 (2004): 125-28. Print.

Berenguer, Beatriz, et al. "Sclerotherapy of Craniofacial Venous Malformations: Complications and Results." Plastic and reconstructive surgery 104.1 (1999): 1-11; discussion 12-5. Print.

Buck II, Donald W, Murad Alam, and John YS Kim. "Injectable Fillers for Facial Rejuvenation: A Review." Journal of Plastic, Reconstructive & Aesthetic Surgery 62.1 (2009): 11-18. Print.

Clark, Richard P, and Craig E Berris. "Botulinum Toxin: A Treatment for Facial Asymmetry Caused by Facial Nerve Paralysis." Plastic and reconstructive surgery 115.2 (2005): 573-74. Print.

Flament, Frederic, et al. "Effect of the Sun on Visible Clinical Signs of Aging in Caucasian Skin." Clinical, cosmetic and investigational dermatology 6 (2013): 221. Print.

Fujimoto, Tomoko, Kazuo Kawahara, and Hiroo Yokozeki. "Epidemiological Study and Considerations of Primary Focal Hyperhidrosis in J Apan: F Rom Questionnaire Analysis." The Journal of dermatology 40.11 (2013): 886-90. Print.

Guttmacher, Alan E, Douglas A Marchuk, and Robert I White Jr. "Hereditary Hemorrhagic Telangiectasia." New England Journal of Medicine 333.14 (1995):

918-24. Print.

Jacovella, Patricio F, et al. "Long-Lasting Results with Hydroxylapatite (Radiesse) Facial Filler." Plastic and reconstructive surgery 118.3S (2006): 15S-21S. Print.

Kablik, Jeffrey, et al. "Comparative Physical Properties of Hyaluronic Acid Dermal Fillers." Dermatologic Surgery 35 (2009): 302-12. Print.

Lacombe, Victor. "Sculptra: A Stimulatory Filler." Facial plastic surgery 25.02 (2009): 095-99. Print.

Mendelson, Bryan, and Chin-Ho Wong. "Changes in the Facial Skeleton with Aging: Implications and Clinical Applications in Facial Rejuvenation." Aesthetic plastic surgery 36.4 (2012): 753-60. Print.

Moraites, Eleni, Olushola Akinshemoyin Vaughn, and Samantha Hill. "Incidence and Prevalence of Hyperhidrosis." Dermatologic clinics 32.4 (2014): 457-65. Print.

Moseley, Timothy A, Min Zhu, and Marc H Hedrick. "Adipose-Derived Stem and Progenitor Cells as Fillers in Plastic and Reconstructive Surgery." Plastic and reconstructive surgery 118.3S (2006): 121S-28S. Print.

Ortonne, Jean-Paul, et al. "Treatment of Solar Lentigines." Journal of the American Academy of Dermatology 54.5 (2006): S262-S71. Print.

Roberts, Wendy E. "Chemical Peeling in Ethnic/Dark Skin." Dermatologic Therapy 17.2 (2004): 196-205. Print.

Russell, Richard. "Sex, Beauty, and the Relative Luminance of Facial Features." Perception 32.9 (2003): 1093-107. Print.

Schick, Christoph H. "Pathophysiology of Hyperhidrosis." Thoracic surgery clinics 26.4 (2016): 389-93. Print.

Smith, Lynnelle, and Kimberly Cockerham. "Hyaluronic Acid Dermal Fillers: Can Adjunctive Lidocaine Improve Patient Satisfaction without Decreasing Efficacy or Duration?" Patient preference and adherence 5 (2011): 133. Print.

Strobl, Walter, et al. "Best Clinical Practice in Botulinum Toxin Treatment for Children with Cerebral Palsy." Toxins 7.5 (2015): 1629-48. Print.

Strutton, David R, et al. "Us Prevalence of Hyperhidrosis and Impact on Individuals with Axillary Hyperhidrosis: Results from a National Survey." Journal of the American Academy of Dermatology 51.2 (2004): 241-48. Print.

Tromovitch, Theodore A, Samuel J Stegman, and Richard G Glogau. "Zyderm Collagen: Implantation Technics." Journal of the American Academy of

Dermatology 10.2 (1984): 273-78. Print.

Warfield, Susanne S. "Estheticians in Dermatology." Dermatologic Therapy 14.3 (2001): 246-54. Print.

CHAPTER 20

References

Allen, John. "Photoplethysmography and Its Application in Clinical Physiological Measurement." *Physiological measurement* 28.3 (2007): R1. Print.

Armstrong, Paul A, et al. "Optimizing Infrainguinal Arm Vein Bypass Patency with Duplex Ultrasound Surveillance and Endovascular Therapy." *Journal of vascular surgery* 40.4 (2004): 724-31. Print.

Aronne, Louis J. "Epidemiology, Morbidity, and Treatment of Overweight and Obesity." *The Journal of clinical psychiatry* (2001). Print.

Arroyo-Johnson, Cassandra, and Krista D Mincey. "Obesity Epidemiology Worldwide." *Gastroenterology Clinics* 45.4 (2016): 571-79. Print.

Avram, Mathew M. "Cellulite: A Review of Its Physiology and Treatment." *Journal of Cosmetic and Laser Therapy* 6.4 (2004): 181-85. Print.

Cordts, Paul R, and Teddie S Gawley. "Anatomic and Physiologic Changes in Lower Extremity Venous Hemodynamics Associated with Pregnancy." *Journal of vascular surgery* 24.5 (1996): 763-67. Print.

Currie, Ph J, et al. "Continuous-Wave Doppler Echocardiographic Assessment of Severity of Calcific Aortic Stenosis: A Simultaneous Doppler-Catheter Correlative Study in 100 Adult Patients." *Circulation* 71.6 (1985): 1162-69. Print.

Eberhardt, Robert T, and Joseph D Raffetto. "Chronic Venous Insufficiency." *Circulation* 111.18 (2005): 2398-409. Print.

Flegal, Katherine M, et al. "Association of All-Cause Mortality with Overweight and Obesity Using Standard Body Mass Index Categories: A Systematic Review and Meta-Analysis." *Jama* 309.1 (2013): 71-82. Print.

Fowkes, FGR, CJ Evans, and Amanda Jane Lee. "Prevalence and Risk Factors of Chronic Venous Insufficiency." *Angiology* 52.1_suppl (2001): S5-S15. Print.

Gloviczki, Peter, et al. "The Care of Patients with Varicose Veins and Associated Chronic Venous Diseases: Clinical Practice Guidelines of the Society for Vascular Surgery and the American Venous Forum." *Journal of vascular surgery* 53.5 (2011): 2S-48S. Print.

Heller, Jennifer. "Treatment of Chronic Venous Insufficiency." *Supplement to Endovascular Today* (2011): 12-15. Print.

Cosmeceuticals for Cellulite. Seminars in cutaneous medicine and surgery. 2011. WB Saunders. Print.

Katsogridakis, Yiannis L, et al. "Veinlite Transillumination in the Pediatric Emergency Department: A Therapeutic Interventional Trial." *Pediatric emergency care* 24.2 (2008): 83-88. Print.

Diagnosis of Chronic Venous Disease of the Lower Extremities: The "Ceap" Classification. Mayo Clinic Proceedings. 1996. Elsevier. Print.

Krysa, J, GT Jones, and AM Van Rij. "Evidence for a Genetic Role in Varicose Veins and Chronic Venous Insufficiency." *Phlebology* 27.7 (2012): 329-35. Print.

Lee, Amanda J, et al. "Lifestyle Factors and the Risk of Varicose Veins: Edinburgh Vein Study." *Journal of clinical epidemiology* 56.2 (2003): 171-79. Print.

Matarasso, Alan, and Tracy M Pfeifer. "Mesotherapy and Injection Lipolysis." *Clinics in plastic surgery* 36.2 (2009): 181-92. Print.

Modrall, J Gregory, et al. "Late Incidence of Chronic Venous Insufficiency after Deep Vein Harvest." *Journal of vascular surgery* 46.3 (2007): 520-25. Print.

Owens, Tracy Martinez. "Morbid Obesity: The Disease and Comorbidities." *Critical care nursing quarterly* 26.2 (2003): 162-65. Print.

Palfreyman, Simon J, Rona Lochiel, and Jonathan A Michaels. "A Systematic Review of Compression Therapy for Venous Leg Ulcers." *Vascular Medicine* 3.4 (1998): 301-13. Print.

Pasquali, Renato, Laura Patton, and Alessandra Gambineri. "Obesity and Infertility." *Current Opinion in Endocrinology, Diabetes and Obesity* 14.6 (2007): 482-87. Print.

Rossi, Ana Beatris R, and André Luiz Vergnanini. "Cellulite: A Review." *Journal of the European Academy of Dermatology and Venereology* 14.4 (2000): 251-62. Print.

Swartz, Melody A. "The Physiology of the Lymphatic System." *Advanced drug delivery reviews* 50.1-2 (2001): 3-20. Print.

Uzuncakmak, Tuğba Kevser, Necmettin Akdeniz, and Ayse Serap Karadag. "Cutaneous Manifestations of Obesity and Themetabolic Syndrome." *Clinics in dermatology* 36.1 (2018): 81-88. Print.